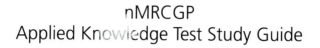

nMRCGP
Applied Knowledge Test Study Guide

WITHDRAWN FROM

D0413422

nMRCGP
Applied Knowledge Test Study Guide

SAMPLE QUESTIONS AND EXPLANATORY ANSWERS

AALIA KHAN
BSc (Hons) MBBS (Dist) DRCOG DFFP MRCGP (Dist)
General Practitioner, London

RAMSEY JABBOUR
BSc (Hons) MBBS DRCOG DFFP DCH MRCGP (Dist)
General Practitioner, London

AND

ALMAS REHMAN
MBBS DFFP DCH MRCGP (Dist)
General Practitioner, London

Radcliffe Publishing
Oxford • New York

Radcliffe Publishing Ltd
18 Marcham Road
Abingdon
Oxon OX14 1AA
United Kingdom

www.radcliffe-oxford.com
Electronic catalogue and worldwide online ordering facility.

© 2008 Aalia Khan, Ramsey Jabbour and Almas Rehman

Aalia Khan, Ramsey Jabbour and Almas Rehman have asserted their right under the Copyright, Designs and Patents Act 1998 to be identified as the author of this work.

All rights reserved. No part of this publication may be reproduced, stored in a retrieval system or transmitted, in any form or by any means, electronic, mechanical, photocopying, recording or otherwise, without the prior permission of the copyright owner.

British Library Cataloguing in Publication Data

A catalogue record for this book is available from the British Library.

ISBN-13: 978 184619 230 2

Typeset by Pindar New Zealand (Egan Reid), Auckland, New Zealand
Printed and bound by Hobbs the Printers Ltd, Southampton, Hampshire, UK

Contents

Preface

As three young, dynamic GPs working in London we realised that there was a dearth of well-written up-to-date MCQ revision guides with satisfactory explanations. Since we all achieved Distinctions in the MRCGP exam we believed we could incorporate our revision notes on hot topics to develop a high-quality contemporary MCQ resource.

The nMRCGP syllabus has been covered in the following four examination papers. These can be attempted individually, or, to allow for focused revision, you may choose to answer questions by subject. These have been grouped together in the index. The explanatory answers have also been fully referenced for your convenience.

We hope you enjoy using this book as much as we enjoyed writing and developing it. We believe that this book will be a vital tool to help you pass the exam with ease and that it will also be a useful reference source in the future to ensure a successful career, based on lifelong learning and patient-centred care.

Finally, we wish you all the very best for the exam.

Dr Aalia Khan
Dr Ramsey Jabbour
Dr Almas Rehman
November 2007

About the authors

Aalia Khan qualified from University College London Medical School in 2000 with a Distinction in Medicine. She trained in obstetrics and gynaecology for three years in London before completing her GP training at the London Deanery. She achieved merits in all four modules of the MRCGP in 2006, gaining a Distinction, and was nominated for the Fraser Rose Medal. She was awarded a gold medal by the Ahmadiyya Muslim Community in recognition of her outstanding achievement in 2006. She is an active member of the RCGP South London Faculty and recently developed her role as South London Tutor for newly qualified GPs. Currently she works as a salaried GP in South London and lives in Surrey.

Ramsey Jabbour currently lives in London and works at the Rood Lane Medical Group in Bishopsgate EC2 with a special interest in Occupational Medicine. He gained a merit in each of the four components of the MRCGP, gaining a Distinction overall, and was nominated for the Fraser Rose Medal in 2006. He undertook his VTS rotation in Maidstone and qualified from University College London Medical School in 2001.

Almas Rehman graduated from The Royal Free Medical School in 2002 knowing that she wanted to be a GP. She went into the Croydon VTS straight after house jobs and was one of the longest serving members! She gained a Distinction in the MRCGP exam in 2006. She is currently working as a salaried GP in a busy, South London practice. She has a special interest in teaching medical students and trainee GPs. At present, she is also the GP mentor for a senior Practice Nurse.

Acknowledgements

Aalia: First of all, Alhamdulillah. Thank you to my husband Mashood and my parents and mother-in-law who supported me in writing this book, especially whilst I was expecting my first child, Safa Maryam. Shazia and Muneeb, you have always supported and prayed for me. Special thanks to Merc, you were a great guinea pig! Ramsey, it was fate that we met at the exam after not seeing each other since medical school, and Almas, I am so grateful you wanted to be part of this too. Well done to all three of us!

Ramsey: Thank you to my partner Ritu for support, humour and music whilst I was writing this book. (*Screamin' Aerosmith now has a whole new meaning!*). To both my parents for guiding and supporting me through my life, and my brother Richard for keeping me sane. To all my friends that I don't know any more, hope to catch up with you soon. Thanks to my GP trainer Mike and VTS tutors for instilling knowledge in me. And finally, thank you to Aalia and Almas and to our continued friendship – here's to enjoying life.

Almas: Jazakallah to my parents and family who have been so patient and understanding, even though you kept trying to distract me Saba. Zakir, sorry, but you'll have to wait a little bit longer for those new car keys. Much love to Shakir, Hina, Ayesha and Sufyaan. Cara, you have my utmost respect – I have no idea how you did this whilst studying for med-school finals! G and Yasmeen, thanks so much for your encouragement and support. We would never have managed to get through those long late-night sessions without your cooking skills, Aalia, and without your boundless enthusiasm Ramsey – so many thanks. Alhamdulillah.

And, of course, a big thank you to Gillian Nineham at Radcliffe Publishing who encouraged us so enthusiastically.

Subject index

Subject	Paper 1 question number	Paper 2 question number	Paper 3 question number	Paper 4 question number
Basic life support	44	28	40	32
Benefits/sick pay	74		63	62
Cardiology	7, 16, 34, 62, 71, 86	1, 20, 33, 41, 55, 68, 74, 86, 90	2, 17, 32, 56, 64, 73	1, 29, 48–52, 61, 67, 78, 83, 89, 100
Cremation forms/ Coroner	24, 66	36	91	2, 91
Dermatology	14, 52–60	31, 57, 84, 89	16, 53, 76, 80, 96	8, 47, 82, 94, 98, 99
Employment/ maternity leave	48, 67		39	42
Endocrinology	25, 50, 89	32, 58, 72	10, 25–30, 59, 97	35, 39, 44, 70, 84, 93
ENT	22	7	88, 95	41, 59
Fitness to drive/fly	9	2	44–51	
Gastroenterology	27, 75–83	6, 30, 54	9, 33, 62, 78	43, 60, 85
Genetics	26	25, 43,73	35, 43, 55	53, 63
Haematology	42	3, 59, 69	7, 75, 93	3–6
Nephrology	45	22, 35, 82	4, 71	87
Neurology	21, 40, 72, 84, 87	29, 44, 77–81	23, 74	11, 34, 71–76

The nMRCGP examination

The membership examination for the Royal College of General Practitioners has undergone a major change. The new curriculum has brought with it a wholly different qualification, called the nMRCGP. It is a mandatory licensing examination for newly qualified GPs, which ensures that they have satisfactorily completed specialist training and are safe to practise independently. The original four-module MRCGP has been replaced by a three-part qualification which includes continual assessment throughout the 3-year vocational training scheme (VTS), which was previously not taken into account when candidates were assessed for membership.

The nMRCGP qualification consists of the following three components.

1 APPLIED KNOWLEDGE TEST (AKT)

A 3-hour, 200 multiple-choice question exam which assesses candidates in the following areas:

* 80% clinical medicine
* 10% critical appraisal and evidence-based clinical practice
* 10% health informatics and administrative issues.

The exam may be taken at any time during the vocational training course. The fully computerised exam takes place three times a year and candidates must sit it at one of the designated exam centres.

2 CLINICAL SKILLS ASSESSMENT (CSA)

This is a competence-based assessment of candidates in which 10-minute consultations with role players will take place under examiner observation. Cases will be based upon clinical disease, e.g.

cardiovascular, respiratory, etc. The criteria for competence must be met for all the assessment areas. The candidate will receive a grade for each of the following areas.

- Primary-care management
  - being able to diagnose and manage problems seen in primary care.
- Problem-solving skills
  - having a structured approach to making decisions, targeted history taking and examinations, relevant use of investigations and using available data to manage a patient.
- Comprehensive approach
  - a holistic approach to managing patients, taking psychosocial aspects into consideration; being aware of risk factors and medical co-morbidities.
- Person-centred care
  - being patient-centred, taking steps to ensure that the patient has understood; seen to be using patient-centred consultation models, asking the patient's opinion.
- Attitudinal aspects
  - a non-judgemental, professional approach to the problem with evidence of good ethical consideration.
- Clinical practical skills
  - competent in physical examinations and the use of common instruments.

3 WORKPLACE-BASED ASSESSMENT (WPBA)

The WPBA is the continual assessment part of the exam. Throughout the VTS, the trainees will undergo 6-monthly progress reviews, results of which will be held in the trainee's portfolio. These assessments and reviews will again be competency based. The following twelve areas have been identified from the core curriculum statement 'Being a General Practitioner'.

- Communication skills/consultation skills
- Practising holistically
- Data gathering and interpretation

- Diagnosis/making decisions
- Clinical management
- Managing medical complexity
- Primary-care administration and information management and technology
- Working with colleagues and in teams
- Community orientation
- Maintaining performance, learning and teaching
- Maintaining an ethical approach to practice
- Fitness to practise

The trainee will be expected to collect pieces of evidence such as case-based discussions and feedback from senior colleagues and patients to support judgements about his or her progress.

You can access further information at www.rcgp.org.uk

Tips on passing the exam

APPLICATION

Check the RCGP website for application details and apply well in time. Remember to budget for the examination fees. www.rcgp.org.uk

PREPARATION

Start preparing in good time. We think that 3 months' preparation is more than adequate for the AKT. Begin by making a note of challenging consultations, either those that you did not feel confident about or those in which you had to look things up. This is a good method of identifying areas of weakness.

Do as many multiple-choice questions as you have the energy to do as this will prepare you for the style and standard of questions. Time yourself to avoid being rushed in the exam. Developing a study group is an excellent way to help increase your knowledge, learn up-to-date guidelines, discuss difficult questions and, importantly, receive support.

Targeted revision is the key; do not get bogged down by the minutiae. Do not try to learn the entire syllabus, but do refer to the RCGP website which will give you an idea of the scope of subjects being examined. We have compiled the following list of resources that we found helpful while preparing for the exam. Much has also been summarised in the answers sections.

USEFUL RESOURCES

Books
Oxford Handbook of General Practice/Clinical Medicine/Clinical Surgery
British National Formulary
Evidence Based Medicine
Clinical Evidence

Publications
British Medical Journal
Journal of Royal College of General Practitioners
British Heart Foundation leaflets
Drugs and Therapeutics Bulletin
Pulse/GP/Doctor magazines

Guidelines/websites
www.rcgp.org.uk
www.eguidelines.co.uk
www.nice.org.uk
www.bhf.org.uk
www.sign.ac.uk
www.brit-thoracic.org.uk
www.dh.gov.uk
www.ffprhc.org.uk
www.rcplondon.ac.uk
www.rcog.org.uk
www.gpnotebook.co.uk
www.dermnet.com
www.emedicine.com
www.bashh.org
www.bash.org.uk

ON THE DAY

Remember to be well rested, i.e. no late-night cramming sessions. Arrive in good time for the exam, since rushing will only stress you unnecessarily. Latecomers will not be admitted. Don't forget your paperwork, which includes your candidate number, and also photographic identification.

It is essential that you visit the examination centre website before sitting the exam, details of which are on the college website. A computer-based tour and demonstration run of the exam are available so that you can familiarise yourself with the procedure, which requires a degree of computer literacy. Mastering this is an added hurdle, don't let it count against you on the day.

READ THE QUESTION – twice if necessary! Answer every question as there is no negative marking. You may be rushed for time, and every year there is a significant number of candidates who fail to complete the exam. Do not dwell on difficult questions for too long; leave them and come back to them at the end.

We realise that most of this advice is obvious but hope that it will serve you well as a quick reminder close to the exam!

Paper 1

Choose the most likely diagnosis from the list below for each clinical scenario (in Questions 1 to 5). Options may be used once, more than once or not at all.

a Simple back pain
b Pott's disease
c Myeloma
d Metastatic bone disease
e Osteoporosis
f Ankylosing spondylitis
g Abdominal aortic aneurysm
h Cauda equina syndrome
i Fibromyalgia
j Spondylolisthesis
k Osteomalacia

1 A 38-year-old woman presents with a 3-month history of lower back pain and generalised morning stiffness. She also complains of numbness and tingling in both feet, urinary frequency and frequent headaches.

2 A 23-year-old man complains of a 2-year history of back pain which is worse in the mornings. He also complains of a red, painful eye.

3 A 32-year-old man complains of a 2-week history of lower back pain after he helped a friend move house. It does not radiate anywhere, and feels like a spasm-type pain. It worsens with bending. On examination there is limited spinal movement.

4   A 68-year-old man presents with a 6-month history of constant backache and weight loss. He also complains of nocturia and frequency.

5   You visit an 89-year-old housebound woman complaining of non-specific back pain. She gets up from her chair with great difficulty to meet you and you notice a waddling gait.

6   Which one statement is not true about Henoch-Schonlein Purpura (HSP)?
   a   The rash is mainly over the buttocks and extensor surfaces.
   b   HSP can be associated with abdominal pain caused by toxic megacolon.
   c   The platelet count is normal.
   d   HSP is more common in boys.
   e   HSP typically occurs after an upper respiratory tract infection.

7   Which one of the following is not true about aortic regurgitation?
   a   It is associated with a collapsing pulse.
   b   It may cause visible neck pulsations.
   c   A diastolic murmur is auscultated.
   d   Sufferers do not require prophylactic antibiotics against endocarditis.
   e   It is associated with Ehler's–Danlos syndrome.

8   Which one of the following is not part of the recommended British Thoracic Society CURB-65 pneumonia score?
   a   Mini mental test score <8/10
   b   Respiratory rate >30 breaths/minute
   c   Heart rate >100 beats/minute
   d   Systolic blood pressure <90mmHg
   e   Age >65 years

9 According to Driver and Vehicle Licensing Agency (DVLA) guidelines, which one of the following does not necessitate stopping driving a car?

   a Myocardial infarction 3 weeks ago

   b Coronary angioplasty 4 weeks ago

   c Seizure-free for 6 months

   d A single episode of amaurosis fugax 4 weeks ago

   e Pacemaker insertion 5 days ago

10 Which of the following is not assessed when determining the International Prostate Symptom Score (IPSS)?

   a Double voiding

   b Urgency

   c Frequency

   d Dysuria

   e Straining to void

11 Drugs that cause dyspepsia include all of the following except which one?

   a Selective serotonin reuptake inhibitors (SSRIs)

   b Calcium antagonists

   c Bisphosphonates

   d Tetracyclines

   e Beta blockers

12 Risk factors for suicide include all of the following except which one?

   a A previous history of deliberate self-harm

   b Increasing age

   c The summer months

   d Lack of employment

   e Divorced men

13 A 78-year-old male presents with a gritty, watery, red, right eye. You notice his lower eyelashes are turned in. What is the diagnosis?

    a Viral conjunctivitis

    b Entropion

    c Iritis

    d Exotropia

    e Allergic conjunctivitis

14 According to the British National Formulary (BNF), what treatment is recommended for cellulitis?

    a Co-amoxiclav

    b Phenoxymethylpenicillin and Flucloxacillin

    c Flucloxacillin

    d Amoxycillin and Flucloxacillin

    e Benzylpenicillin

15 Which of the following statements is true regarding osteoporosis?

    a Peak bone mass occurs in the fourth decade of life.

    b Premenopausal hip bone loss does not occur in women.

    c Male bone loss occurs around the sixth decade.

    d Genetic factors account for 80% of the peak bone mass.

    e Smoking increases bone mass.

16 Beta blockers of proven benefit in heart failure include all of the following except which one?

    a Atenolol

    b Bisoprolol

    c Carvedilol

    d Metoprolol

    e Nebivolol

17 At what age would you expect a child to draw a 'cross'?

a 1 year

b 2 years

c 3 years

d 4 years

e 5 years

18 The following are true about British Thoracic Society (BTS) guidelines on pulmonary emboli (PE) except which one?

a A negative D-dimer reliably excludes a PE.

b Isotope scanning is the recommended initial radiological investigation for non-massive PE.

c All patients with a possible PE need to have their probability assessed and recorded.

d D-dimer tests should only be considered following assessment of clinical probability.

e Computed tomography pulmonary angiography (CTPA) is the recommended initial radiological investigation for non-massive PE.

19 Which one statement is true about Practice-based Commissioning (PBC)?

a Universal coverage means that primary care trusts have to provide all practices with information on how to understand and organise PBC.

b Practices should be able to redirect at least 90% of any freed-up resources.

c GPs will need to contract directly with providers for new services.

d Practices must work together to implement PBC.

e PBC is a locally enhanced service (LES).

20 Which of the following statements regarding combined oral contraceptive pill (COCP) use according to the Faculty of Family Planning July 2006 guidance is true? Choose one statement.

   a Women can start taking the COCP up to and including day 5 of their cycle without the need for additional contraceptive protection.

   b Women taking liver enzyme inducing drugs can rely on the efficacy of COCP containing 20 mcg ethinylestradiol.

   c There is evidence of additional weight gain due to COCP use.

   d Unscheduled bleeding during COCP use is a measure of lowered efficacy.

   e If a woman is >14 days post-partum, is not breastfeeding and has not resumed her menstrual cycle she may start the COCP as if she is amenorrhoeic, i.e. start it at any time if reasonably certain she is not pregnant.

21 Which one of the following standardised tests is not recommended by NICE for use when formally assessing cognition to diagnose dementia?

   a 7-Minute Screen

   b Mini Mental State Examination (MMSE)

   c Mental Alternation Test

   d General Practitioner Assessment of Cognition (GPCOG)

   e 6-Item Cognitive Impairment Test (6-CIT)

22 A 23-year-old man complains of a painful right ear with a foul-smelling discharge. There is a past history of traumatic perforation on the same side from a diving accident. In addition, you notice a lower motor neuron facial nerve palsy. What is the diagnosis?

   a Chronic otitis externa

   b Cholesteatoma

   c Otitis media with effusion

   d Malignant otitis externa

   e Osteatoma

23 Concerning the influenza vaccination, which of the following statements is true?

a The vaccine changes each year depending on the prevalent strains.

b It is a live vaccine.

c It is recommended for all working-age people.

d It is contraindicated in HIV-positive people.

e It is safe in those with egg allergy.

24 Which of the following does not need to be referred to the Coroner?

a Death in a road traffic accident

b Death where doctor has attended the patient within the last 10 days

c Patient dying of mesothelioma

d Patient dying within 24 hours of hospital admission

e Patient dying in police custody

25 A 29-year-old female presents with increased irritability, diarrhoea and 3-kg weight loss in 3 months. On examination she has a rapid, regular pulse, sweaty palms and a mild tremor. She also has a small goitre. Bloods taken show the following. What is the diagnosis?

Thyroid stimulating hormone (TSH) 0.03mU/L (0.3–5.0mU/L)
Free thyroxine (FT4)   34.8pmol/L(9–25pmol/L)
Free triiodothyronine (FT3)   15pmol/L   (3–9mol/L)
Auto antibodies to TSH receptor   Positive

a Hashimoto's thyroiditis

b Grave's disease

c Myxoedema

d Toxic multi-nodular goitre

e De Quervain's thyroiditis

26 Which one of the following is an example of autosomal dominant inheritance?

a Marfan's syndrome

b Cystic fibrosis

c Sickle-cell disease

d Haemochromatosis

e Tay-Sach's disease

27 A 21-year-old man presents with fatigue and pallor. On further questioning, he states his stools have become jet black. You notice perioral pigmentation. What is the diagnosis?

a Familial adenomatosis polyposis coli

b Peutz–Jegher's syndrome

c Ulcerative colitis

d Crohn's disease

e Peptic ulcer disease

Using the table below, match up the serological results with the correct diagnosis (in Questions 28 to 32). Each result may be used once, more than once or not at all.

	HBsAg	HBeAg	Anti-HBe	Anti-HBc IgG	Anti-HBc IgM	Anti-HBs
a	+++	+	-	+	-	-
b	-	-	-	-	-	+
c	-	-	+/-	+	-	+
d	+	+/-	+/-	+	+++	-
e	+	-	+	+	-	-

Abbreviations:
HBsAg   Hepatitis B surface antigen
HBeAg   Hepatitis B envelope antigen
Anti-HBe   Antibody to Hepatitis B envelope antigen
Anti-HBc IgG   IgG Antibody to Hepatitis B core antigen
Anti-HBc IgM   IgM Antibody to Hepatitis B core antigen
Anti-HBs   Antibody to Hepatitis B surface antigen
HBV   Hepatitis B Virus

28 Acute HBV infection

29 High-infectivity HBV carrier

30 Low-infectivity HBV carrier

31 Past infection with HBV

32 Immunised against HBV

33 Which one of the following is not a recognised complication of cystic fibrosis?
  a Diabetes insipidus
  b Pyloric stenosis
  c Meconium ileus
  d Infertility
  e Short stature

34 Which one of the following statements is not true?
  a Beta blockers are less effective than Angiotensin Converting Enzyme (ACE) inhibitors at reducing blood pressure.
  b Angiotensin II receptor antagonists are associated with an increased risk of myocardial infarction.
  c Evidence suggests that home blood-pressure monitoring is not to be encouraged.
  d Treating hypertension with a combination of a beta blocker and a diuretic can increase the risk of a patient developing diabetes.
  e Statins are to be used in patients with a 10-year cardiovascular risk >20%.

35 A 3-day-old breast-fed baby presents with a 24-hour history of jaundice. On examination, he is afebrile and looks well. What is the most likely diagnosis?
  a Infection
  b Haemolysis
  c Breast-milk jaundice
  d Polycythaemia
  e Biliary atresia

36 Which one of the following is not true of Dupuytren's contracture?

    a May occur bilaterally.

    b Caused by thickening of the carpal tunnel fascia.

    c May occur in the feet.

    d Can run in families.

    e May affect women.

37 Which of the following is defined as a detailed review and statistical analysis of data pooled from a number of studies to reach a result?

    a Cohort study

    b Meta-analysis

    c Retrospective study

    d Systematic review

    e Qualitative analysis

38 A recommended treatment for *Trichomonas vaginalis* infection is:

    a Metronidazole 400mg tds for 10 days

    b Amoxicillin 500mg tds for 5 days

    c Metronidazole 400mg bd for 5 days

    d Ciprofloxacin 500mg po stat

    e Azithromycin 1g po stat

39 In the drug treatment of panic disorder the medication of choice is:

    a Citalopram

    b Olanzapine

    c Diazepam

    d Amitriptylline

    e Mirtazapine

40 A 45-year-old man presents with a left-sided headache centred around his eye, which is watering and red. He states that he has had this before and attacks last around 1 hour, usually after he has had wine with a meal. What is the acute treatment of choice?

a Paracetamol

b Intramuscular Diclofenac

c Oral sumatriptan

d Subcutaneous sumatriptan

e Verapamil

41 A 56-year-old hypertensive gentleman treated with perindopril and nifedipine presents with pitting oedema. What would be the best course of action?

a Start frusemide

b Start bendrofluazide

c Stop perindopril

d Increase perindopril

e Stop nifedipine

42 A 26-year-old asymptomatic Greek gentleman has some routine blood tests. The results are as follows. What is the diagnosis?

Haemoglobin	11.7g/dL	(13.5–18g/dL)
Mean corpuscular volume (MCV)	61.1fl	(80–100fl)
Platelet count	179×10^9/L	(150–400×10^9/L)
White cell count	7.1×10^9/L	(4–11×10^9/L)
Serum iron	20.5mcmol/L	(14–32mcmol/L)
Serum ferritin	90mcg/L	(30–233mcg/L)

a Iron deficiency

b Beta thalassaemia trait

c Sickle-cell disease

d Ulcerative colitis

e Vitamin B12 deficiency

43 What is the Quality and Outcomes Framework (QOF) target for total serum cholesterol in secondary prevention after a transient ischaemic attack (TIA) or stroke?

a ≤3.0mmol/L

b ≤3.5mmol/L

c ≤4.0mmol/L

d ≤4.5mmol/L

e ≤5.0mmol/L

44 How long should the rescuer take in looking, listening and feeling for breaths in a victim, before assuming that he/she is not breathing and commencing cardiopulmonary resuscitation?

a 5 seconds

b 10 seconds

c 15 seconds

d 20 seconds

e 25 seconds

45 Which is the most common type of renal stone?

a Calcium phosphate

b Xanthine

c Calcium oxalate

d Struvite

e Cysteine

46 A 60-year-old male suddenly loses his vision. The retina looks like a 'stormy sunset'. What is the diagnosis?

a Occlusion of the central retinal artery

b Occlusion of the central retinal vein

c Vitreous haemorrhage

d Retinal detachment

e Branch occlusion of central retinal vein

47 A 65-year-old woman presents with weight loss, malaise, pain on brushing her hair and pain in her upper arms when getting out of her chair. What is not included in your differential diagnosis?

a Fibromyalgia

b Hyperthyroidism

c Tuberculosis

d Osteoporosis

e Polymyalgia rheumatica

48 A receptionist who has worked at the surgery for 5 years informs you that she is pregnant and wants to take maternity leave. How much leave is she entitled to?

a 12 weeks' ordinary maternity leave

b 12 weeks' ordinary maternity leave and 12 weeks' additional maternity leave

c 15 weeks' ordinary maternity leave and 15 weeks' additional maternity leave

d 26 weeks' ordinary maternity leave and 15 weeks' additional maternity leave

e 26 weeks' ordinary maternity leave and 26 weeks' additional maternity leave

49 Which of the following statements is true of varenicline?

a It should be started on the day smoking is stopped.

b Bupropion is more effective.

c NICE draft guidance 2007 advises that varenicline should not be available on the NHS.

d It is a partial agonist at the nicotine receptor.

e It is administered transdermally via a skin patch.

50 A 58-year-old type-2 diabetic presents for his 6-monthly review. He takes metformin. His blood pressure reading is 140/80mmHg and he has 1+ microalbuminuria. What is your management?

a Verapamil

b Bendroflumethiazide

c Ramipril

d Atenolol

e Increase metformin

51 Which one of the following is not a diagnostic criterion for Kawasaki's disease according to NICE?

a Cervical lymphadenopathy >10mm diameter

b Fever >5 days

c Bilateral conjunctivitis

d Cervical lymphadenopathy >15mm diameter

e Strawberry tongue

Choose the most likely diagnosis from the list below for each clinical scenario (in Questions 52 to 60). Options may be used once, more than once or not at all.

a Tinea incognito

b Acne rosacea

c Granuloma annulare

d Psoriasis

e Basal cell carcinoma

f Dermatitis herpetiformis

g Scabies

h Pompholyx

i Erythema multiforme

j Tinea corporis

k Warts

l Eczema

m Ichthyosis

n Keratoderma blennorrhagica

o Pyoderma gangrenosum

p Pityriasis rosea

q Necrobiosis lipoidica

r Erysipelas

s Lyme disease

t Lichen planus

u Lichen sclerosus

v Venous ulcer

w Erythema nodosum

x Malignant melanoma

y Molluscum contagiosum

z Pityriasis versicolor

52 A 35-year-old lady with ulcerative colitis presents with a rapidly enlarging painful ulcer on her lower leg after a minor knock.

53 A 12-year-old boy is bought in by his parents. He has not stopped itching for over a week and his sleep is disturbed. The rest of the family is now affected.

54 A 26-year-old female presents with a spreading rash over her shin; this was diagnosed by another GP as eczema and has been treated with increasing strengths of steroid creams. It decreased the redness but now the rash has spread.

55 A 25-year-old female presents with a rash in her perineal area. It consists of small discrete lesions approximately 3mm in diameter that are dome-shaped and umbilicated. Squeezing the lesions produces a creamy discharge.

56 A 20-year-old man presents with a ring-like lesion on the back of his hand, the border is elevated with a central involuted area. He is a known diabetic.

57 A 38-year-old male presents with itchy shins. On examination, scale-like lesions are present.

58 A 35-year-old teacher presents with a fever and cold. He has also noticed an expanding target-like patch on his forearm. He has recently been on holiday to Eastern Europe where he partook in forest walks.

59 A 25-year-old female presents with tender pink nodules on her shins; she has recently had co-trimoxazole for a urinary tract infection.

60 A 23-year-old gentleman presents with a pustular rash on the soles of his feet. He also has painful finger joints and dysuria. He states this all occurred since he was treated for conjunctivitis 4 days ago.

61 Which one of the following statements is not true about fibrosing alveolitis?
   a A productive cough may be a presenting symptom.
   b Honeycomb shadows are a late sign on chest x-ray.
   c Antinuclear antibodies and rheumatoid factor are present in 10% of patients.
   d Fine end-inspiratory crepitations are heard on auscultation (Velcro crepitations).
   e Erythrocyte sedimentation rate (ESR) tends to be elevated.

62 Which one of the following medications does not worsen heart failure?
   a Diclofenac
   b Lithium
   c Phenytoin
   d Verapamil
   e Prednisolone

63 According to the Childhood Immunisation Schedule (September 2006), at what age does a child receive three injections on one visit?
   a 2 months
   b 3 months

c   4 months

d   12 months

e   13 months

64 Which of the following is not a notifiable disease?

a   Viral hepatitis

b   Relapsing fever

c   Malaria

d   Schistosomiasis

e   Acute encephalitis

65 One of The British Hypertension Society criteria for the diagnosis of pre-eclampsia is:

a   Diastolic BP reading of >80mmHg and proteinuria on 2 occasions

b   Diastolic BP reading of >90mmHg and proteinuria on 1 occasion

c   Diastolic BP reading of >95mmHg and no proteinuria on 2 occasions

d   Diastolic BP reading of >100mmHg and no proteinuria on 1 occasion

e   Diastolic BP reading of >110mmHg and proteinuria on 1 occasion

66 What part of the cremation form is completed by a doctor appointed by the Home Office acting as a medical referee undertaking the final check of the forms?

a   Part B

b   Part C

c   Part D

d   Part E

e   Part F

67 The following are true except which one?

a All clinical staff must attend basic life-support training every 18 months.

b Practices have to undergo significant event analysis regularly.

c All staff should receive basic life support training every 36 months.

d Appraisals for staff should take place every 6 months.

e Patient surveys must be undertaken every year.

68 Which one of the following statements is not true of gout?

a Affects men predominantly

b Usually peripheral distribution

c Due to disorder of pyridoxine metabolism

d Characterised by hyperuricaemia

e May result in tophi formation

69 What is the definition of specificity of a screening test?

a The true positive rate

b The negative predictive value

c The false positive rate

d The true negative rate

e The false negative rate

70 Which one of the following is not true about mucolytics in the treatment of chronic obstructive pulmonary disease (COPD)?

a N-acetylcysteine is an example of a mucolytic.

b Mucolytics do not significantly reduce COPD exacerbations if used.

c N-acetylcysteine can induce anaphylaxis.

d NICE guidelines advise that mucolytics should be considered in COPD patients with a chronic cough productive of sputum.

e Mucolytics can be prescribed on a NHS FP-10 prescription.

71 According to NICE hypertension guidelines 2006, what is the most appropriate treatment option for a 45-year-old Chinese man on ramipril with a sustained blood pressure of >160/90mmHg?

a Change to amlodipine

b Add in amlodipine

c Change to bendrofluazide

d Add in atenolol

e Change to losartan

72 A 64-year-old gentleman who suffered from shingles 3 months ago presents with a burning pain over the same area. It is not responsive to simple analgesia. What is your treatment of choice?

a Diclofenac

b TENS machine

c Amitriptyline

d Gabapentin

e Aciclovir

73 Which of the following is not a recommended investigation when assessing benign prostatic hypertrophy?

a Serum PSA

b Renal ultrasound

c Digital rectal examination

d Urinalysis

e Serum urea and electrolytes

74 What form would you issue for a terminally ill patient to receive benefits?

a Med 4

b Med 6

c Med 7

d RM 7

e DS 1500

Choose the most likely diagnosis from the list below for each clinical scenario presented (in Questions 75 to 83). Any option can be used once, more than once, or not at all.

a Gastro-oesophageal reflux disease (GORD)
b Peptic ulcer
c Pancreatitis
d Inferior myocardial infarction (MI)
e Acute cholecystitis
f Biliary colic
g Ureteric colic
h Femoral hernia
i Appendicitis
j Diverticulitis
k Acute epididymitis
l Testicular torsion
m Lead poisoning
n Inguinal hernia
o Intussusception
p Volvulus
q Colorectal cancer
r Diabetic keto-acidosis
s Perforated duodenal ulcer
t Gastroenteritis
u Aortic abdominal aneurysm

75 A 36-year-old male smoker presents with epigastric pain worsened by food. He has lost weight and is pale on examination.

76 An 18-year-old male presents with worsening abdominal pain, constipation and loss of appetite over the past month. The pain is felt all over his abdomen but more concentrated in his right iliac fossa. Rectal examination is normal, his haemoglobin level is 10.4g/dL (13–18g/dL) and basophilic stippling is seen on the blood film. He works in the furniture restoring trade.

77 A 26-year-old man presents with a sudden onset of severe scrotal pain. On examination he has tender hard left testicle that is higher than the right. Lifting the testis does not relieve the pain.

78 A 64-year-old smoker with a history of angina presents with epigastric pain and vomiting. He is hypotensive, pale and sweaty. His abdomen is soft and some bowel sounds are present.

79 A 26-year-old woman with mild pyrexia presents with a 2-day history of abdominal pain, vomiting and loss of appetite. She is particularly tender on examination in her right iliac fossa which is also reproduced on pressing the left iliac fossa.

80 A 65-year-old man presents with increased bowel frequency, blood per rectum, left iliac fossa pain and a mild pyrexia.

81 A 36-year-old female presents with groin pain and vomiting. On examination you notice a hard round swelling just lateral to her pubic tubercle that is extremely tender to touch.

82 A 35-year-old female presents with right upper quadrant (RUQ) and shoulder tip pain. She appears restless and mildly jaundiced. The pain is worse on palpation of the RUQ on deep inspiration. She is apyrexial.

83 A 56-year-old presents with fever, tachycardia, hypotension and epigastric pain, radiating to the back. He has a known history of gallstones. On examination he has a firm, tense abdomen and no bowel sounds.

84 Which of the following beta blockers is likely to be beneficial in the treatment of essential tremor?

a Atenolol

b Metoprolol

c Sotalol

d Propranolol

e Nadolol

85 Which one of the following statements is true of pelvic inflammatory disease (PID)?

   a It is the only cause of female infertility.

   b It is caused by chlamydia in around 50% of cases.

   c Chlamydia and gonorrhoea infection cannot co-exist.

   d The cardinal feature is vaginal discharge.

   e Menstrual irregularities occur in about 5% of cases.

86 Which one of the following statements is true about Q-waves on an ECG?

   a They are always indicative of an MI.

   b They are only significant if they are more than 0.04s in width and greater than 2mm in depth.

   c They are only significant if they are more than 0.12s in width and greater than 2mm in depth.

   d They directly precede a T-wave.

   e If present, they indicate a recent infarct.

87 According to NICE guidelines, for how long after a transient ischaemic attack (TIA) or stroke should patients be on a combination of aspirin and dipyridamole?

   a 6 months

   b 12 months

   c 18 months

   d 24 months

   e Not at all

88 A 75-year-old asthmatic lady presents with a sore tongue and mouth. On examination there are white creamy patches adherent to her buccal mucosa. What would be your further management?

   a Oral co-amoxiclav

   b Ferrous sulphate supplementation

   c HIV testing

   d Amphotericin

   e Aciclovir

89 A 45-year-old gentleman presents with a fatigue, polyuria and polydipsia. He also describes muscle weakness. On examination you notice a high blood pressure. The only abnormality in his blood tests is a low serum potassium level. What is the diagnosis?

a Cushing's disease

b Conn's syndrome

c Phaeochromocytoma

d Diabetes insipidus

e Addison's disease

90 What skill would you expect a 3-year-old child to have recently acquired?

a Kicking a ball

b Feeding self with a spoon

c Using a knife and fork to eat

d Removing own clothes

e Walking upstairs unaided

91 Carpal tunnel syndrome is diagnosed clinically by:

a Symptoms reproduced when the wrist is forcibly palmar flexed and pressure applied to the median nerve

b Symptoms reproduced by tapping directly on the ulnar nerve

c Symptoms reproduced by forcibly extending the wrist and applying pressure to the median nerve

d Extending both wrists for 30 seconds to reproduce symptoms

e Detecting the presence of hypothenar muscle wasting.

92 According to the BNF, what is the first-line treatment for atypical pneumonia?

a Amoxicillin for 7 days

b Clarithromycin for 7 days

c Penicillin V for 7 days

d Cephalexin for 7 days

e Amoxicillin for 5 days

93 Which one of the following is not a contraindication for intrauterine contraceptive device (IUCD) insertion?

a Wilson's disease

b Immunosuppression

c History of ectopic pregnancy

d Uterine cavity distortion

e Trophoblastic disease

Which of the following Sections under the Mental Health Act 1983 would apply in each scenario (in Questions 94 to 100)? Options may be used once, more than once or not at all.

a Section 4

b Section 8

c Section 112

d Section 2

e Section 135

f Section 36

g Section 136

h Section 3

i Section 12

j Section 115

k Section 7

l None at all

94 A schizophrenic patient has stopped taking his medication, resulting in a deterioration of his condition. He refuses voluntary admission.

95 A known homeless man presents smelling of alcohol, stating he is suicidal. He shows you some minor cut marks on his wrists. He claims he is being controlled by an outside influence and is having difficulty sleeping because he can hear voices. He refuses hospital admission.

96 A concerned relative of a 72-year-old man who has recently lost his wife contacts you. You visit him and deem him to be suicidal. He states 'he wants to die and nothing will stop him doing it today'. On examination he displays a flat affect and has a dishevelled appearance. There are a number of paracetamol boxes next to him and there is no one that can be with him. He refuses admission and is angry that you have come.

97 A 56-year-old woman has barricaded herself in her home; you are concerned, as the last time you saw her she had neglected her appearance and smelt of urine. She refuses entry to you as she fears she is possessed by the devil and only bad things will happen.

98 You receive a report from the local Out-of-Hours service regarding a 78-year-old demented woman who is cared for by her daughter. It states that their visiting doctor noticed a number of bruises over her body. You are concerned of ongoing abuse by the daughter. However, she has refused you entry to see the patient.

99 An 18-year-old has recently threatened schoolchildren with a knife, claiming he is controlled by an external force that is compelling him to do so. He denies drug abuse. He refuses admission, stating, 'You are preventing justice, I am the chosen one.'

100 A teenager is found wondering naked on the street, shouting and spitting at passers-by. He does not seem intoxicated, but is clearly responding to voices.

Answers Paper 1

1 i

2 f

3 a

4 d

5 k

Fibromyalgia is a musculoskeletal condition of unknown cause. It is characterised by pain which is usually axial; specific tender sites in the body – diagnosed if more than 11/18 sites are involved; generalised morning stiffness; fatigability and other associated symptoms such as abdominal pain, headache and urinary frequency. Most common in women aged 40–50 years (90% of sufferers). Management, after the diagnosis has been made by excluding other causes, focuses on supportive treatment, reassurance that no serious pathology exists and information. Sometimes referral to a pain clinic or rheumatology is required.

Ankylosing spondylitis is a seronegative arthropathy; 2.5 times more common in males; can run in families, and in 95% of cases is HLA B27 positive. It is characterised by chronic back pain and morning stiffness in young people. Associated symptoms include hip/knee arthritis, iritis, osteoporosis, psoriaform rashes, colitis/Crohn's and plantar fasciitis. Remember the bamboo spine on x-ray caused by fusion and squaring of the vertebrae. Management includes exercise, NSAIDs, referral to rheumatology or other specialities as appropriate.

Simple back pain is the most common scenario. There is often a history of heavy lifting. Sufferers are around 20–55 years old, otherwise well with no sign/symptom of inflammatory disease. Management includes reassurance, avoiding bed rest and keeping as active as possible. There is no need to x-ray routinely. Simple analgesia, e.g.

paracetamol/NSAIDs, is usually sufficient. Physiotherapy referral for symptom relief and postural exercises is an option.

So many red flags in one question can only mean malignancy. Weight loss and constant backache are clues, as is the patient's age. Also can you guess the primary? Most commonly they are kidney, lung, prostate, breast and thyroid. With nocturia and frequency you wouldn't go wrong with prostate cancer. Remember to read all the words in a question, they are there for a reason.

Osteomalacia is not uncommon in the housebound elderly who are at great risk of being malnourished. The waddling gait and difficulty getting out of the chair are due to proximal muscle weakness in the pelvic and shoulder girdles. Management will include a vitamin-D supplement (800 IU/day), dietary advice, social input, etc.

6 b

The underlying cause of Henoch-Schonlein Purpura (HSP) is a widespread immune mediated vasculitis which typically presents with a purpuric rash over the buttocks and extensor surfaces after an upper respiratory tract infection, more often in boys. There may be associated arthritis, nephritis, and bowel intussusception with malaena. Periorbital oedema, testicular inflammation and rarely, central nervous involvement causing fits or coma can occur.

7 d

Aortic regurgitation is commonly caused by rheumatic heart disease, endocarditis, aortic dissection and congenital defects. Rarely, it is associated with Ehler's–Danlos, Osteogenesis Imperfecta and Marfan's disease. Symptoms include dyspnoea and palpitations. Characteristic signs include a collapsing pulse (water hammer); visible neck pulsations (Corrigan's sign); head nodding (De Musset's sign), and visible capillary pulsations (Quincke's sign). The murmur is a mid-diastolic murmur. Valve replacement should be done early to prevent further impairment of left ventricular function. Prophylactic antibiotics are required against endocarditis.

8 c

The CURB-65 community-acquired pneumonia score has been developed to aid clinicians in deciding who needs to be admitted to hospital.

C – **C**onfusion (mental test score <8)
U – **U**rea level >7mmol/L
R – **R**espiratory rate >30 breaths/min
B – **B**lood pressure (systolic BP <90mmHg; diastolic BP <60mmHg)
65 – Age >**65** years

One point is awarded for each criterion. A score of 1 or 2 requires assessment in hospital and a score of 3 or 4 requires admission, www. brit-thoracic.org.uk

9 b

Patients are fit to drive a week after coronary angioplasty.

10 d

The IPSS is an objective measure of symptoms to grade severity (mild, moderate and severe) and is very helpful when assessing symptoms of benign prostatic hypertrophy (nocturia, double voiding, urgency, frequency, straining) in deciding whether a referral to the urologist is warranted. More information on www.eguidelines.co.uk

11 e

12 c

Higher rates have been documented in the spring and autumn but not summer. Other risk factors include having a psychiatric or physical illness, alcohol abuse, drug addiction and social isolation.

13 b

Senile entropion affects the lower eyelid only and treatment includes lubrication and surgery. More recently Botox® is being used as an alternative but is only a temporary measure.

14 b

15 d

Peak bone mass occurs in the third decade of life. Premenopausal hip bone loss does occur, around the fourth or fifth decade. Male bone loss starts around the fifth decade. Smoking REDUCES peak bone mass. Genetic factors account for 80% of the peak bone mass. Reference: www.gpnotebook.co.uk

16 a

Atenolol and propranolol are not cardioselective beta blockers.

17 d

A 3-year-old child is able to draw a circle; a 4-year-old is able to draw a cross and a 5-year-old can draw a triangle.

18 b

According to BTS guidelines for pulmonary emboli (2003) all patients need to have their probability assessed and recorded. D-dimer testing should only be carried out on those patients that need it and who have had a good-quality chest x-ray. A negative D-dimer test reliably excludes a PE. CTPA is the imaging of choice for non-massive PE.

19 a

PBC is a directly enhanced service (DES) which will be more successful if a number of surgeries are involved with implementation, but this is not a mandatory point. More information on PBC can be found on the government website: http://www.dh.gov.uk/en/Policyandguidance/ Organisationpolicy/Commissioning/Practice-basedcommissioning/ index.htm

20 a

The COCP should be started on day 1 of the menstrual cycle. However, it can be started up to and including day 5 of the cycle without the need for additional protection. Only COCP containing at least 50mcg ethinylestradiol are reliable enough for women taking liver enzyme inducing drugs. In fact, it is best practice to advise them to use contraception unaffected by liver enzyme inducing drugs if it is needed long term. There is no evidence of additional weight gain due to COCP use. Unscheduled bleeding whilst on the COCP is not a measure of efficacy if not associated with missed pills/vomiting within 2 hours of pill taking/severe diarrhoea or drug interactions. If a woman is >21 days post-partum, is not breastfeeding and has not resumed her menstrual cycle, she may start the COCP at any time. Reference: http://www.ffprhc.org.uk/admin/uploads/FirstPrescCombOral ContJan06.pdf

21 c

Reference: http://guidance.nice.org.uk/cg42

22 b

A cholesteatoma is usually visualised as a pearly white ball in the pars flaccida. It can increase in size, invading nearby structures and may lead to hearing loss, headache, vertigo, facial nerve palsy and a cerebral abscess.

23 a

24 b

Any suspicious death needs to be reported to the Coroner. Others include: death that occurs at home without a doctor having seen the patient within the last 14 days; death that occurs within 24 hours of hospital admission; death during surgery or before recovering from an anaesthetic; and death that occurs due to industrial reasons.

25 b

Grave's disease is an autoimmune disorder caused by auto-antibodies to the TSH receptor, resulting in stimulation and overriding of the normal negative feedback axis controlling T4 and T3 production. A similar auto-immune process occurs in the soft tissue of the orbit, hence the ophthalmological manifestation seen in Grave's – proptosis, exophthalmos and ophthalmoplegia. www.gpnotebook.co.uk

26 a

Marfan's syndrome is an example of autosomal dominant inheritance. Other examples include Huntingdon's disease, adult polycystic kidney disease and neurofibromatosis type 1. Cystic fibrosis, Tay-Sach's and sickle-cell disease are recessive conditions.

27 b

Peutz–Jegher's syndrome is an autosomal dominant disorder characterised by muco-cutaneous pigmentation and intestinal polyps. Patients have an increased risk of developing cancer and so it is important to include these patients in a surveillance programme.

28 d

29 a

30 e

31 c

32 b

IgM antibody is produced as an immediate response whilst IgG is a memory response. Therefore IgM will only be present in a patient currently infected with HBV. Vaccinated individuals will exhibit Anti-HBs whilst a patient who has been infected in the past will make antibody to the envelope and core antigens as well. A low infectivity carrier will not exhibit HBeAg.

33 a

Recognised complications of cystic fibrosis include bronchiectasis, pneumothorax, both Aspergillus and Pseudomonas infections and respiratory failure. Others include: pancreatic insufficiency; pyloric stenosis; meconium ileus; failure to thrive; short stature; gallstones; infertility and rectal prolapse.

34 c

Refer to NICE Hypertension guidelines, June 2006.

35 c

Physiological jaundice is caused by hepatic immaturity and excessive destruction of foetal red cells. Jaundice within the first 24 hours of life tends to indicate serious pathology such as infections, ABO incompatibility, and Rhesus haemolytic disease of the newborn or red-cell abnormalities such as spherocytosis. Jaundice presenting between day 2 and day 7 is usually physiological or due to breast feeding (though this is not a reason to stop breast feeding). Prolonged jaundice after seven to ten days can be due to hypothyroidism, biliary atresia and galactosaemia.

36 b

Caused by thickening of the palmar fascia.

37 b

Meta-analysis is a statistical re-analysis of pooled data from studies identified by systematic reviews to reach a more accurate conclusion. Pooling the data increases the overall power, providing a better chance of producing a statistically significant result. It is most commonly used to assess the clinical effectiveness of healthcare interventions. www.evidence-based-medicine.co.uk

38 c

Also Metronidazole 2g stat orally. BASSH guidelines state that there is evidence that *T. vaginalis* is associated with preterm labour and low birthweight. Also it may enhance HIV transmission. Reference: http://www.bashh.org/guidelines

39 a

NICE 2007 guidance: The evidence suggests that cognitive behavioural therapy has the most long-lasting beneficial effect. Where medical therapy is needed, a selective serotonin re-uptake inhibitor (SSRI) licensed for use in panic disorder is the treatment of choice.

40 d

According to the British Association for the Study of Headache (BASH) 2007 guidelines, drug treatment for an acute cluster headache is ALWAYS necessary. First-line treatment is 6mg sumatriptan subcutaneously. BASH also recommends giving 100% oxygen to stop an attack. Analgesics, ergotamine and oral triptans are of no use in the acute treatment of cluster headache. Verapamil is used for prophylaxis first line and alcohol must be avoided. www.bash.org.uk

41 e

Side-effects of nifedipine include headache, flushing, dizziness and pitting oedema.

42 b

The red blood cells are low in both haemoglobin and in microcytic but both the serum iron and ferritin are normal. Treatment with iron is not warranted. Haemoglobin electrophoresis will show a raised Hb-A2 +/- raised Hb-F.

43 e

The total serum cholesterol level of a patient after a TIA or stroke for QOF targets should be ≤5.0mmol/L. It is important to read the question as the British Hypertension Society (BHS) guidelines state total cholesterol should be ≤4.0mmol/L. BHS guidelines also state statins should be commenced for primary prevention in people with high blood pressure who have a 10-year risk of developing cardiovascular disease (CVD) of 20%, unlike the National Service Framework which is based on a 10-year risk of developing coronary heart disease (CHD) of 30% and above. The BHS guidelines are much tighter and reflect the importance of stroke prevention as well (CVD risk of 20%≈CHD risk of 15%). Reference for up-to-date QOF targets: http://www.nhsemployers.org/primary/primary-890.cfm

44 b

Reference: www.resus.org.uk. You must look this up for the current guidelines.

45 c

Calcium stones are the most common and oxalate is the commonest type, followed by uric acid, struvite and then cysteine. Infection with *Proteus sp.* results in staghorn calculi caused by struvite.

46 b

Central retinal vein occlusion causes painless loss of vision and is more common in the elderly. It is associated with hypertension and chronic glaucoma. On examination, the retina exhibits a 'stormy sunset' appearance due to haemorrhages near engorged vessels. Peripheral vision is better repaired than central vision. Laser coagulation has been shown to be beneficial in some cases.

47 b

Differential diagnoses of polymyalgia rheumatica make up a long list and include many systemic/vasculitic/infective/bone diseases. Malignancy is always in the mix as well. However, hypothyroidism rather than hyperthyroidism is more implicated here.

48 e

From 1 April 2007 all expectant mothers are entitled to 52 weeks of maternity leave in total, made up of 26 weeks' ordinary leave and 26 weeks' additional leave. This may not all be paid leave, though. Currently statutory maternity pay is payable for 39 weeks. Reference: www.direct.gov.uk

49 d

Varenicline is a new oral smoking cessation product. It should be started a week before the agreed stopping smoking date and has been approved in NICE 2007 draft guidance. Studies have shown that varenicline is twice as effective as bupropion. It is a partial agonist at the nicotine receptor. Binding alleviates the symptoms of craving and withdrawal, as well as reducing both the rewarding and reinforcing effects of nicotine.

50 c

The HOPE study concluded that cardiovascular deaths in diabetic patients with high blood pressure started on ACE inhibitors were reduced beyond that of just lowering the blood pressure. ACE inhibitors are also known to slow the progression of renal disease in both types 1 and 2 diabetes. The Heart Outcomes Prevention Evaluation (HOPE) study. *New England Journal of Medicine.* 2000; **342**: 145–53.

51 a

The diagnostic criteria for Kawasaki's disease (NICE 2007, *Feverish illness in children*) are a fever for 5 days >39 °C and at least four of the following: change in mucus membranes (e.g. injected pharynx, cracked lips or strawberry tongue); bilateral conjunctival injections; polymorphous rash; change in peripheral extremities (e.g. oedema, erythema or desquamation) or cervical lymphadenopathy (≥1 **node**, ≥**1.5cm** in size). www.nice.org.uk

52 o

53 g

54 a

55 y

56 c

57 m

58 s

59 w

60 i

Tinea incognito is due to the misdiagnosis and hence mistreatment of a tinea infection. The doctor believes the rash to be dermatitis and treats it with a topical steroid leading to a spreading fungal infection. Steroids should be stopped and standard anti fungal treatment should be initiated.

Ichthyosis can either be inherited or acquired. Acquired may be secondary to hypothyroidism, HIV, sarcoid, cancer, lymphoma or medication, e.g. hydroxyurea.

61 c

Fibrosing alveolitis is a disease characterised by an increase in inflammatory cells and lung fibrosis. It can be associated with other connective tissue disorders, autoimmune thyroid disease and ulcerative colitis. Patients present with a dry cough, exertional dyspnoea, weight loss and malaise. Signs include clubbing and fine end-inspiratory crepitations (Velcro crepitations). Chest x-ray shows a honeycomb pattern as a late sign. Antinuclear antibodies and rheumatoid factor are present in 35% of patients. ESR is usually raised. Lung biopsy may be needed for diagnosis and staging. Immunosuppresion with steroids is the mainstay of treatment.

62 c

Medications contraindicated in heart failure include non-steroidal anti-inflammatory drugs, steroids, lithium and calcium channel blockers such as verapamil.

63 c

Vaccines received at 4 months of age: DTP/IPV/Hib, Men C, PCV.

D – diphtheria, T – tetanus, P – pertussis, IPV – polio, Hib – Haemophilus influenzae type b, PCV – Pneumococcal conjugate vaccine. www.immunisations.nhs.uk

64 d

Reference: http://www.hpa.org.uk/infections/topics_az/noids/noidlist.htm

65 e

The second criterion is a diastolic BP reading of >90mmHg and proteinuria on 2 occasions.

66 e

The Home Office requires an independent doctor to perform a final check of the cremation form and complete Part F. Part D is issued if a post mortem is performed. When an inquest is opened into a death, the Coroner issues Part E.

67 d

All non-clinical practice staff must undergo an annual appraisal. Reference: http://www.nhsemployers.org/primary/primary-890.cfm

68 c

Due to disorder in purine metabolism.

69 d

The proportion of all those who test negative and do not have the disease over the total number of people who do not have the disease.

70 b

NICE COPD guidelines 2004 advise that mucolytics can be trialled in patients and, if they are effective, can be used as maintenance therapy. N-acetylcysteine is an example of an effective mucolytic that has been shown to reduce the number of exacerbations; however; it can induce anaphylaxis. Mucolytics can be prescribed on a NHS FP-10 prescription.

71 b

NICE Hypertension Guidelines 2006 recommend that patients younger than 55 years be treated with an ACE inhibitor as first line, with the addition of a calcium channel blocker or a diuretic if further treatment is necessary.

72 c

Post herpetic neuralgia can last for months to years after an episode of shingles. The most effective treatment is a tricyclic antidepressant.

73 b

An ultrasound of the kidneys is unnecessary if serum creatinine is measured. Also consider post-void residual volume measurement and flow rates (these may not be accessible from primary care). Reference: www.eguidelines.co.uk

74 e

A DS 1500 form is for patients who are terminally ill. A doctor is legally required to state a patient is incapable of working if the sickness exceeds 7 days, including the weekend, for Statutory Sick Pay purposes. The doctor must examine the patient on the day or the day before issuing a Med 3, for a period of 1 month initially. A Med 5 is used either when the issuing doctor has not examined the patient but has a written report from another doctor regarding the patient's illness, or the examination took place on a previous occasion. A Med 4 is usually requested by the Department of Works and Pensions (DWP) after 28 weeks of incapacity to confirm the nature of the illness and allows for an independent medical opinion on fitness to work (the Personal Capability Assessment). It is used in assessing patients for state benefits. A RM7 is used to request an independent opinion sooner if the practitioner is in any doubt about the patient's situation. A Med 6 is completed and sent to the DWP if an accurate diagnosis is not disclosed on the Med 3, 4 or 5.

75 b

76 m

77 l

78 d

79 i

80 j

81 h

82 f

83 c

In the diagnosis of acute appendicitis, Rovsing's sign is positive: when pressing on the left iliac fossa, greater tenderness is elicited in the right iliac fossa.

Murphy's sign is positive in acute cholecystitis: tenderness is elicited when the hand is placed under the right costal margin and the patient is asked to inhale. This is because the inflamed gallbladder descends and comes into contact with the examining hand. The same manoeuvre is negative in the left upper quadrant.

84 d

Reference: www.clinicalevidence.com

85 b

PID is an upper genital tract infection, most commonly a complication of chlamydia infection in around 50% of cases. Of course different STIs can coexist. The complication rate for PID is high, around 25% after only a single episode of PID. PID is thought to be a common cause of female infertility. The commonest presentation is with lower abdominal pain/tenderness. Infertility may be the presentation with PID being diagnosed retrospectively. Menstrual irregularities occur in about 25% of cases.

86 b

On an ECG, Q-waves are thought to be non-significant if small and present in the left ventricular leads. If the Q-wave is >0.04 seconds in width and >2mm in depth, it is thought to be pathological. Although indicative of infarction, there is no correlation with the age of an infarct. They directly precede the R-wave.

87 d

According to NICE guidelines – Vascular disease May 2005 – patients should be on a combination of aspirin and dipyridamole for 2 years after a TIA or stroke.

88 d

Side-effects of inhaled steroids include candidal infections of the oropharynx, dysphonia, bruising, adrenal suppression, and in children can cause stunting in growth. These are more pronounced with higher doses and poor technique. Patients should be advised to gargle after using their steroid inhaler.

89 b

75% of cases are due to an adrenal adenoma requiring surgical treatment.

90 c

Children can kick a ball and undress themselves by the age of 4 years. They are able to feed themselves with a spoon and walk upstairs unaided by the age of 2 years. They can use a knife and fork to eat by the age of 3 years.

91 a

Phalen's test (forcibly palmar flexing the wrist and applying pressure to the median nerve), Tinel's test (tapping on the median nerve directly to reproduce symptoms), the wrist *flexion* test (*flexing* both wrists for 30 seconds to reproduce symptoms) and *thenar* muscle wasting are all diagnostic signs of carpal tunnel syndrome.

92 b

Clarithromycin or erythromycin are to be used for atypical pneumonia.

93 c

Other contraindications include: recent sexually transmitted disease not fully investigated or treated; severe anaemia; pregnancy; unexplained uterine bleeding; genital malignancy; pelvic inflammatory disease and copper allergy. Cautions include: valvular heart disease; nulliparity; young age; scarred uterus; menorrhagia; history of ectopic pregnancy; tubal surgery; fertility problems and diabetes. Reference: www.bnf. org

94 h

95 l

96 a

97 e

98 j

99 d

100 g

Under the Mental Health Act 1983, the following Sections can be used only if voluntary admission is impossible, the patient has a mental disorder and requires inpatient admission and treatment, and he or she poses a risk to self or others.

Section 2. Compulsory admission for 28 days for assessment. It is not renewable and the patient can appeal within 2 weeks via a Mental Health Tribunal. Two medical recommendations are required to apply the Section, one doctor must be Section 12 approved.

Section 3. Admission for treatment for 6 months or less; can be renewed indefinitely. The exact mental disorder must have been diagnosed. The patient has a right to appeal.

Section 4. Emergency admission for assessment lasting 72 hours only. The application can be made by the nearest relative or an approved social worker and must be supported by one doctor. The doctor must have examined the patient within the previous 24 hours. A Section 4 can be converted into a Section 2 after 72 hours by applying to a Section 12 approved doctor if further assessment is required.

Section 115. An Approved Social Worker (ASW) is granted powers of entry and inspection to the premises of a mental health patient when there is concern that the patient is not receiving proper care or is a threat to self or others.

Section 135. An ASW is granted the power to search and remove an adult where there is reasonable cause to suspect that a mental health patient is not receiving proper care; is being ill-treated or neglected; is unable to care for him- or herself; or is a threat to self or others.

Section 136. Gives power to police officers to intervene if the adult is in a public place, to remove them to a place of safety, e.g. a hospital casualty department.

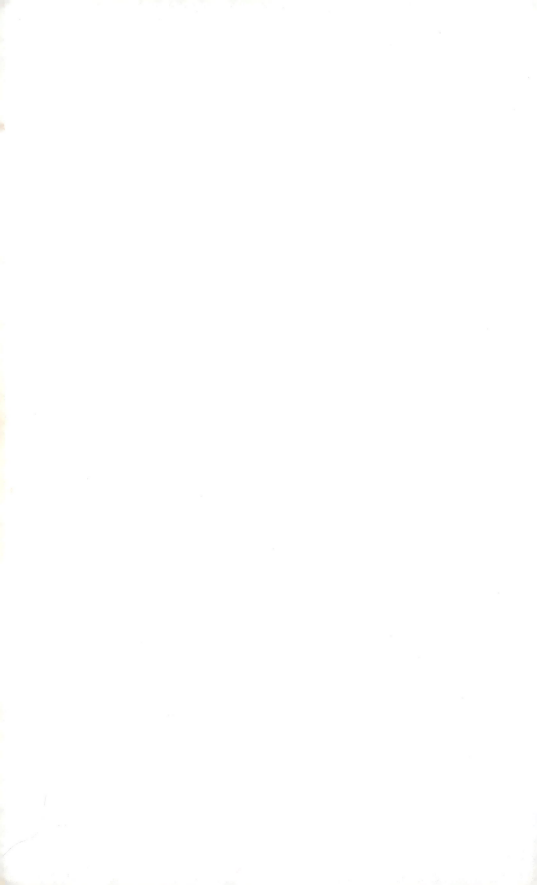

Paper 2

1 If a patient is taking frusemide for heart failure, what is the next medication to introduce according to NICE heart failure guidelines?

a Ramipril

b Digoxin

c Losartan

d Atenolol

e Spironolactone

2 According to leading airlines and the World Health Organisation, what is the minimum requirement of haemoglobin to fly?

a 7.0g/dL

b 7.5g/dL

c 8.0g/dL

d 6.5g/dL

e 8.5g/dL

3 Which one of the following statements is not true about immune thrombocytopenic purpura (ITP)?

a ITP may be chronic or acute.

b Antiplatelet immunoglobulin (IgG) antibodies are present.

c Anti-nuclear antibodies (ANA) are positive in approximately 40% of patients.

d Splenomegaly can be palpable.

e Retinal haemorrhage is common.

4   According to the Childhood Immunisation Schedule (September 2006), when should the first Meningitis C vaccine be given?

   a   2 months

   b   3 months

   c   4 months

   d   12 months

   e   13 months

5   How much does the Department of Health pay practices per patient for producing a plan which sets out how services will be organised for Practice-based Commissioning (PBC), i.e. Direct Enhanced Services (DES) component 1?

   f   90p

   g   95p

   h   85p

   i   80p

   j   £1.00

6   Which one of the following is not a recognised side-effect of proton pump inhibitors?

   a   Pigmented tongue

   b   Flatulence

   c   Abdominal distension

   d   Insomnia

   e   Diarrhoea

7   Concerning the treatment of acute otitis media, which one of the following statements is true?

   a   Antibiotics are always needed.

   b   Co-Amoxiclav is the first line treatment of choice.

   c   Children under two with fever or vomiting may require antibiotic treatment.

   d   A delayed prescription is of no use.

   e   Analgesia does not help.

8 According to the British National Formulary (BNF) how many weeks should a non-steroidal anti-inflammatory drug (NSAID) be tried before switching to another due to failure of its anti-inflammatory effect?

   a 2
   b 3
   c 4
   d 5
   e 6

9 Concerning depression in patients post-myocardial infarction, which one of the following statements is true?

   a There is no link between patients who have suffered a myocardial infarction and depression.
   b Sertraline is safe and effective post-MI.
   c There is no evidence that treatment of depression improves survival.
   d Tricyclic antidepressants are the treatment of choice.
   e We should avoid asking patients about symptoms of depression as the realisation could make it worse.

From the list below, select the most appropriate treatment for each clinical scenario (in Questions 10 to 19). Each treatment option may be used once, more than once or not at all.

   a Chloramphenicol eye drops
   b Sodium cromoglicate eye drops
   c Fusidic acid eye drops
   d No treatment
   e Oral aciclovir
   f Non-steroidal anti-inflammatories
   g Dexamethasone eye drops
   h Pilocarpine eye drops
   i Aciclovir eye ointment
   j Pad the eye and analgesia
   k Eyelid hygiene

10 A 40-year-old welder complains of red watery eyes. On examination, there is no foreign body. He has notable blepharospasm.

11 A 25-year-old contact-lens wearer presents with pain and blurred vision in his left eye. Examination shows a green lesion under blue light when the eye is instilled with fluorescein dye.

12 A 3-year-old child presents with a 4-day history of a sticky right eye, especially in the morning. On examination, yellow discharge can be seen on the eye lashes and slight redness of the affected eye.

13 A 70-year-old hypertensive man presents with a sudden, painless localised redness to his right eye. The vision is not impaired.

14 A 45-year-old man present with a sudden onset of pain in his left eye. He has blurred vision. On examination the eye is watering and the pupil is noted to be irregular with circumcorneal redness.

15 A 26-year-old female presents with bilateral red, watery and itchy eyes. On examination, the eyes are red with 'cobblestones' visible under the upper eyelids.

16 A 60-year-old female presents with itchy eyes and redness of the lid margins. On examination, there are scales present on the eyelashes.

17 A 30-year-old HIV-positive patient presents with a rash and pain around his left eye. His complains of tingling on the tip of his nose. On examination, the eye is red with a small irregular pupil.

18 A 65-year-old man notes a sudden blurring of his vision which gets worse during the evening. The pain in his eye also worsens. On examination, the oval-shaped pupil is fixed and dilated.

19 A patient presents with a dull ache in the right eye which is also tender to touch. On examination, the sclera looks blue below engorged vessels.

20 Which one of the following is not useful in diagnosing peripheral vascular disease?

a Clinical examination

b Dopplers for ankle brachial pressure index

c Angiography

d Thyroid function tests

e Serum cholesterol

21 Carpal tunnel syndrome is not more common in which one of the following conditions?

a Pregnancy

b Hyperthyroidism

c Acromegaly

d Sarcoidosis

e Amyloidosis

f Diabetes mellitus

22 According to the Health Protection Agency (HPA) guidelines for management of uncomplicated urinary tract infection (UTI) in adult women, when it is appropriate to prescribe an antibiotic empirically, i.e. no need to send a urine culture?

a Two symptoms of UTI present AND no vaginal discharge/ irritation

b Negative nitrites, positive leucocytes on urine dipstick

c Negative nitrites and leucocytes, positive blood and protein on urine dipstick

d Three or more symptoms of UTI present AND no vaginal discharge/irritation

e Nitrites, leucocytes, blood, protein all negative on urine dipstick

23 Which of the following steroid-base creams is the strongest?

    a Trimovate®

    b Eumovate®

    c Betnovate®

    d Hydrocortisone

    e Dermovate®

24 The following statements are true regarding the use of beta blockers in heart failure, except which one?

    a Beta blockers should be considered in all patients with heart failure who are able to take them.

    b Beta blockers are contraindicated in all patients with chronic obstructive pulmonary disease.

    c Beta blockers of proven benefit in heart failure include carvedilol and bisoprolol.

    d In trials, the use of beta blockers in heart failure resulted in a relative risk reduction in mortality of around 35%.

    e It may take up to 6 months for the beneficial effects of beta blockers on left ventricular function to appear.

25 Which one of the following is not a cause of tall stature?

    a Congenital adrenal hyperplasia

    b Kleinfelter's syndrome

    c Hypothyroidism

    d Soto's syndrome

    e Hyperthyroidism

26 According to the January 2007 NICE guidelines, what is the first-line pharmaceutical treatment for menorrhagia if no histological or structural abnormality is suspected and the woman has no preference for hormonal or non-hormonal treatment?

    a Tranexamic Acid

    b Levonorgestrel releasing intrauterine system

    c Mefenamic Acid

    d Norethisterone

    e The oral combined contraceptive pill

27 What drug may be prescribed as a heroin substitute?

   a Paracetamol

   b Buprenorphine

   c Codydramol

   d Ibuprofen

   e Migraleve

28 Regarding the use of an automatic external defibrillator (AED), for how many minutes should cardiopulmonary resuscitation continue before the AED rechecks the rhythm?

   a 1 minute

   b 2 minutes

   c 3 minutes

   d 4 minutes

   e 5 minutes

29 The November 2006 NICE guidelines for dementia define mild cognitive impairment as:

   a Cognitive decline expected for a person's age

   b Cognitive decline greater than expected for a person's age and education level which affects activities of daily living

   c Cognitive decline greater than expected for a person's age and education level which does not notably affect activities of daily living

   d Cognitive decline in those with previous learning disabilities

   e None of the above.

30 Gallstones are associated with which one of the following?

   a Ulcerative colitis

   b Irritable bowel syndrome

   c Crohn's disease

   d Males

   e Low BMI

31 Which of the following statements is false concerning acne rosacea?

   a May present with recurrent facial flushing.

   b Rhinophyma is a complication.

   c Affects women more than men.

   d Comedones are a feature.

   e More common in fair-skinned people.

32 What type of primary thyroid tumour commonly affects the under-40s?

   a Medullary adenocarcinoma

   b Follicular adenocarcinoma

   c Papillary adenocarcinoma

   d Lymphoma

   e Anaplastic carcinoma

33 According to NICE hypertension guidelines, if a patient is on three medications, e.g. ramipril, bendrofluazide and amlodipine, and the blood pressure is still >150/90mmHg, which one is not a recognised treatment option?

   a Further diuretic treatment

   b Addition of an alpha receptor antagonist

   c Addition of a beta blocker

   d To consider specialist advice

   e To consider hospital admission

34 Which hearing test would be most appropriate for a 6-month-old child?

   a Brain stem evoked potential

   b Otoacoustic emission

   c Threshold audiometry

   d Speech discrimination testing

   e Distraction testing

35 What is the annual incidence of uncomplicated urinary tract infection (UTI) in women in the UK?

a   5%

b   10%

c   15%

d   20%

e   25%

36 Who is permitted to complete and sign Part C of the cremation form?

a   Partner of GP signing Part B

b   Wife of GP signing Part B

c   Another GP in the same practice

d   A hospital doctor with no connection to the doctor signing Part B

e   Brother of deceased patient who is a doctor

37 Which one of the following is true about corticosteroids in asthma?

a   Patients should gargle after using inhaled steroids.

b   They act within 2 hours.

c   Decrease only tracheal mucosal inflammation.

d   High-dose oral steroids should be used as a regular treatment option.

e   Will tend to cause osteoporosis.

38 According to NICE guidelines, the treatment of choice for a newly diagnosed patient with schizophrenia is:

a   Olanzapine

b   Clozapine

c   Stelazine

d   Sulpiride

e   Levomepromazine

39 A healthcare assistant has joined your practice. Which immunisation should you offer him?

  a Varicella

  b Hepatitis A

  c Pneumococcus

  d BCG

  e Meningitis C

40 According to April 2005 WHO Selected Practice Recommendations for Contraceptive Use, which of the following statements regarding missed pills is false?

  a If a woman misses three or more 30–35mcg ethinylestradiol pills in week 3 (days 15–21) of the pill packet, she should omit the pill-free interval; i.e. a new pack should be started without the 7-day break.

  b Barrier methods or abstinence should be used for 7 days if three or more 30–35mcg ethinylestradiol pills are missed.

  c Two pills can be taken on the same day, or even at the same time, depending on when the woman remembers.

  d The woman requires emergency contraception if she has missed one or two 30–35mcg ethinylestradiol pills at any time.

  e The most recent missed pill should be taken as soon as the woman remembers.

41 What is the commonest causative organism of infective endocarditis?

  a *Pseudomonas aeruginosa*

  b *Staphylococcus aureus*

  c *Streptococcus viridans*

  d *Streptococcus pneumoniae*

  e *Mycoplasma pneumoniae*

42 In the Quality and Outcomes Framework (QOF), points are awarded for all of the following except which one?

a   Legible records.

b   A reliable system to ensure that home-visit requests are recorded and doctors can action them.

c   Patients are able to access a receptionist for at least 45 hours per week.

d   Patients can access the out-of-hours with no more than two phone calls.

e   Recording the smoking status of patients aged 21–75 years.

43 Select the true statement regarding genetic and risk factors for osteoporosis:

a   The risk of osteoporosis is greater in obese women.

b   The B polymorphism of the vitamin D receptor gene is under-represented in women with low postmenopausal bone density.

c   Peak bone mass in adulthood is not controlled by genetic factors.

d   Exhibiting polymorphism for the Type I collagen gene (COLIA I) will increase the risk of osteoporotic fractures.

e   A family history of osteoporosis does not increase risk.

44 Which Angiotensin Converting Enzyme inhibitor has been shown to reduce recurrent stroke risk even in patients with normal blood pressure?

a   Ramipril

b   Enalapril

c   Perindopril

d   Lisinopril

e   Losartan

45 Concerning malaria prophylaxis, which of the following statements is true?

   a Antimalarial prophylaxis is 100% effective.

   b Antimalarial prophylaxis is best taken before meals.

   c If a patient suffers from a fever above 38 °C and a 'flu like illness within 1 year of returning from a malaria zone, it is important to seek medical advice.

   d There is no need to use other preventative measures, e.g. DEET/long sleeves.

   e Chloroquine is the best choice.

Match the following diagnoses with the clinical scenarios below (in Questions 46 to 53). Each option may be used once, more than once or not at all.

   a Osteochondritis dissecans

   b Anterior cruciate ligament rupture

   c Bi-partite patella

   d Iliotibial band syndrome

   e Medial shelf syndrome

   f Fat pad syndrome

   g Patella tendonitis

   h Posterior cruciate ligament rupture

   i Medial collateral ligament rupture

   j Meniscal tear

   k Patella dislocation

   l Osteoarthritis

   m Septic arthritis

   n Patella-femoral mal-alignment

   o Sickle crisis

   p Psoriatic arthropathy

   q Gout

   r Pseudogout

   s Rheumatoid arthritis

t Reiter's

u Osgood Schlatter's disease

46 A 20-year-old footballer presents with a swollen knee which occurred after he was tackled. He felt a 'popping' sensation, and since then describes instability on that leg. He feels his knee 'giving way' and a sense of weakness. Lachman's test is positive.

47 A 45-year-old keen jogger presents with pain along his medial knee joint line. He states he has a vague ache throughout the day and a mild swelling of the knee especially after exercise. He describes the sensation of his knee joint locking.

48 A 15-year-old boy presents with knee ache worse after activity, and a mild knee effusion. He states he has a feeling of locking where he has to flick the knee to straighten it, especially after sitting for a long time. Knee x-rays show a white lesion approximately 0.2cm in the knee joint.

49 A 32-year-old keen walker attends with pain just below his patella, at the insertion of the tendon. It is worse while walking, jumping and going down a flight of stairs.

50 A 13-year-old boy who is on all his sports teams at school presents with pain and tenderness over his tibial tuberosity on his right leg. He states it is worse after playing sports.

51 A 26-year-old female presents with aching around the patella. There is no point tenderness and she states it is worse on sitting for long periods. She also states that the pain is worse on climbing stairs. You notice on examination she has flat feet and weak quadriceps.

52 A 76-year-old gentleman presents with an acutely swollen painful right knee. X-ray shows calcification of the articular cartilage. A joint aspirate shows positively bi-refringent crystals.

53 A 28-year-old man who has recently started training for the London Marathon presents with pain over the lateral aspect of the knee. He states it has worsened since his training commenced.

54 Symptoms consistent with irritable bowel syndrome (IBS) include all of the following except which one option?

  a Abdominal pain

  b Pain relief with defecation

  c Pain associated with increased bowel motions

  d Fever

  e Mucus in stool

55 What is the normal QRS complex duration on an ECG?

  a <0.12s

  b <0.18s

  c <0.05s

  d <0.25s

  e <0.2s

56 Choose one incorrect statement regarding non-specific urethritis (NSU):

  a May be asymptomatic

  b Is treated with doxycycline 100mg bd for 7 days

  c Can be due to chlamydia infection in up to 50% of cases

  d Can be due to Neisseria gonorrhoea infection in up to 30% of cases

  e Requires contact tracing.

57 The best treatment for scalp seborrhoeic dermatitis is:

  a Calcipotriol

  b Ketoconazole shampoo

  c Hydrocortisone

  d Dithranol

  e Emollients

58 A city broker presents with a feeling of being tired all the time. Blood test results reveal the following. What is your management?

Thyroid-stimulating hormone (TSH) 6.2 mU/L (0.3–5.0 mU/L)
Free thyroxine (FT4)   11.0 pmol/L (9–25 pmol/L)

a Start treatment with thyroxine 25 micrograms/day.

b Check thyroid peroxidase antibodies.

c Start carbimazole treatment.

d Start treatment with thyroxine 50 micrograms/day.

e Repeat thyroid function tests in 3 months' time.

59 A 64-year-old lady complains of back pain that is constant in nature. She has also been feeling increasingly tired and constipated. Blood test results show the following. What is the diagnosis?

Alkaline phosphatase	100IU/L	(30–200IU/L)
Calcium	3.2mmol/L	(2.05–2.6mmol/L)
Phosphate	1.9mmol/L	(0.8–1.5mmol/L)

a Metastasis

b Osteoporosis

c Multiple myeloma

d Sarcoidosis

e Primary hyperparathyroidism

60 Which one of the following statements about bupropion to aid smoking cessation is false?

a The maximum period of treatment is 7–9 weeks.

b Treatment is commenced 1–2 weeks before the target stop date.

c It may increase the risk of seizures.

d It is contra-indicated in bipolar disease.

e Concomitant use of anti-depressants is an absolute contra-indication.

61 Which one of the following is not associated with Down's syndrome?

a Learning difficulties

b Hyperthyroidism

c Cataracts

d Duodenal atresia

e Alzheimer's disease

A screening test for bowel cancer using the detection of faecal occult blood is launched. One thousand people take part. Of the 400 who have cancer, 290 test positive, and 390 people in total test positive. From the list of values below answer the following questions (Questions 62 to 67). Each option may be used once, more than once or not at all.

a 500

b 290/400

c 110

d 290/390

e 80%

f 500/600

g 390

h 1000

i 500

j 290

k 500/610

l 600

m 290/600

n 100

62 What is the positive predictive value (PPV) of the test?

63 What is the negative predictive value (NPV) of the test?

64 What is the sensitivity of the test?

65 What is the specificity of the test?

66 What is the number of false positive results?

67 What is the number of false negative results?

68 Which one of the following statements is false about mitral stenosis?

a The pulses are of normal character.

b Is a systolic murmur.

c Generally has a loud S1 heart sound.

d Can cause peripheral cyanosis.

e Can cause right heart failure.

69 A 32-year-old man presents with gingival hypertrophy and swelling. He complains of fatigue and looks pale with diffuse petechiae. What is the diagnosis?

a Acute Myeloid Leukaemia (AML)

b Acute Lymphocytic Leukaemia (ALL)

c Chronic Lymphocytic Leukaemia (CLL)

d Chronic Myeloid Leukaemia (CML)

e Myelofibrosis

70 A 3-year-old child presents with a fever and a maculo-papular rash. On examination, she has red, watery eyes and whites spots on her buccal mucosa. What is the most likely diagnosis?

a Measles

b Bacterial conjunctivitis

c Rubella

d Roseola infantum

e Varicella zoster

71 A 3-week-old baby boy presents with jaundice associated with pale stools, dark urine and vomiting. On examination, he is afebrile and his weight is on the 25th centile. What is the most likely diagnosis?

a Haemolysis

b Biliary atresia

c Physiological jaundice

d Infection

e Breast-milk jaundice

72 A 38-year-old man presents with high blood pressure unresponsive to medication. He also describes having episodes of palpitations and sweating. Which of the following is the most likely diagnosis?

a Phaeochromocytoma

b Carcinoid

c Hyperthyroidism

d Addison's disease

e Conn's syndrome

73 A couple present for antenatal screening. Both have sickle-cell trait. What is the likelihood of their child having sickle-cell disease?

a 50%

b 40%

c 100%

d 33.3%

e 25%

74 Which statement is not true of the Anglo-Scandinavian Cardiac Outcomes Trial (ASCOT)?

a The trial was stopped early.

b The combination of perindopril and amlodipine was compared with atenolol and a thiazide diuretic.

c The combination of perindopril and atenolol was compared with amlodipine and a thiazide diuretic.

d All patients had hypertension and three other risk factors.

e The combination of medication reduces new-onset diabetes by 30%.

75 What is the background risk of developing pre-eclampsia (i.e. if a pregnant woman has no risk factors)?

a 1 in 1000

b 1 in 2000

c 1 in 250

d 1 in 500

e 1 in 1500

76 A 63-year-old female presents with sudden loss of vision in her left eye. On further questioning, she states she also has been suffering from a 'headache' over that eye, and tenderness while combing her hair. On examination you notice a tender hard left temporal artery and pale optic discs. What is the diagnosis?

a Migraine

b Temporal arteritis

c Arterial embolism

d Sub-dural bleed

e Transient ischaemic attack

Match the following nerve roots to the corresponding reflexes (in Questions 77 to 81). Each option may be used once, more than once or not at all.

a C1
b C2
c C3
d C4
e C5
f C6
g C7
h T1
i T2
j T3
k T4
l L1
m L2
n L3
o L4
p L5
q S1
r S2
s S3

77 Biceps reflex

78 Achilles reflex

79 Brachioradialis reflex

80 Triceps reflex

81 Patellar reflex

82 Which one of the following does not increase the risk of renal stones?

    a Nuts

    b Immobilisation

    c Horseshoe kidney

    d Chocolate

    e Oranges

    f Diuretics

    g Strawberries

    h Beetroot

83 Concerning Hepatitis C virus (HCV) infection, which one of the following statements is true?

    a The UK started to screen blood products for HCV in the 1980s.

    b HCV is most commonly transmitted in the UK by sexual intercourse.

    c There is no treatment.

    d The majority of people will develop acute hepatitis.

    e HCV antibodies take up to 3 months to become detectable.

84 With respect to the treatment of scabies, which one of the following statements is true?

    a Permethrin 1% is first-line treatment of choice.

    b It may take 3 weeks for the itching to subside after successful treatment.

c Malathion needs to be left on for 8–12 hours.

d Malathion should be applied after a hot bath to dry and draw the mites to the surface.

e Treatment should be reserved for infected individuals only, and only on the affected areas.

85 A 2-year-old child is noted to be of short stature. She was solely breast fed until the age of 18 months. On examination, she displays wrist splaying and frontal bossing. What is the most likely cause for this?

a Vitamin A deficiency

b Vitamin B deficiency

c Vitamin C deficiency

d Vitamin D deficiency

e Vitamin E deficiency

86 What 10-year cardiovascular risk level is required prior to commencing a statin for primary prevention?

a 10%

b 15%

c 20%

d 25%

e 30 %

87 According to the British Association of Sexual Health and HIV (BASHH), an acceptable treatment for a pregnant woman with chlamydia is:

a Doxycycline 100mg bd for 7 days

b Erythromycin 500mg qds for 7 days

c Ofloxacin 200mg bd for 7 days

d Azithromycin 2g po stat

e Phenoxymethylpenicillin 500mg qds for 7 days

88 Osteoporosis is associated with which one of the following?

   a Hypothyroidism

   b Type II Diabetes mellitus

   c Patau's syndrome

   d Aspirin use

   e Hyperparathyroidism

89 A 28-year-old man presents with a fever and a hot, tender, indurated, red rash on his cheek. The treatment of choice is:

   a Aciclovir

   b Phenoxymethylpenicillin

   c Flucloxacillin

   d Flucloxacillin and penicillin V

   e Metronidazole

90 Which one of the following statements is not true about coronary artery bypass graft operations?

   a The patient can drive after 2 months.

   b Is an option if anti-anginal medication fails.

   c Is an option if there is left main stem disease.

   d The patient's own saphenous vein can be used.

   e The patient's own internal mammary artery can be used.

91 Gestational hypertension by definition

   a is detected after 30 weeks' gestation

   b is hypertension without proteinuria

   c resolves within 6 months of delivery

   d is hypertension with proteinuria

   e is a blood pressure measurement of $\geq 130/85\text{mmHg}$.

Choose one diagnosis for each clinical scenario below (in Questions 92 to 97). Each option may be used once, more than once or not at all.

   a Pulmonary embolism

   b Pneumothorax

c   Streptococcal pneumonia

d   Asthma

e   Chronic obstructive pulmonary disease

f   Lung cancer

g   Cystic fibrosis

h   Atypical pneumonia

i   Obstructive sleep apnoea

j   Legionella pneumophila

92 A 5-year-old child has been coughing at night for the past 2 weeks. He is afebrile and otherwise well in himself. On examination the chest is clear.

93 A 50-year-old ex-smoker presents with a 4-week history of a cough and a hoarse voice. On examination, there is decreased air entry in the right upper zone and you notice wasting of the small muscles of the hand.

94 A young lady who is on the oral contraceptive pill presents with shortness of breath and pleuritic chest pain. On examination, she is tachypnoeic, afebrile and has no chest signs on auscultation.

95 A tall, slim 20-year-old man presents with shortness of breath and chest pain. On examination, he has a respiratory rate of 28 respirations per minute and there are decreased breath sounds on the left.

96 A 35-year-old businessman presents with a fever and persistent dry cough. On examination his pulse rate is 100 beats per minute. There are right basal coarse crepitations on chest auscultation.

97 A 40-year-old man has recently returned from a holiday in Spain. He is complaining of joint pains, lethargy and cough. On chest auscultation there are left basal crepitations.

98 Concerning live vaccines which one of the following is false?

    a Rubella immunisation should not be administered in pregnancy.

    b When two live vaccines are required, they should either be given simultaneously at different sites or separated by a 3-week interval.

    c Rabies vaccination is an example.

    d Live vaccines should not be given to people with impaired immunity.

    e MMR can be given to HIV-positive patients.

99 Which of the following can be used for the prophylaxis of mountain sickness (unlicensed indication)?

    a Acetazolamide

    b Verapamil

    c Mannitol

    d Atenolol

    e Bendrofluazide

100 Regarding the NHS Bowel Cancer Screening Programme effective from April 2006, which statement is not true?

    a Men and women aged 60–69 years are eligible to participate.

    b Screening will take place every 2 years.

    c GPs will receive a copy of their patients' results.

    d It is anticipated that around 5% of participants will have a positive result and will require further investigation.

    e The pilot programme resulted in an uptake of 50%.

Answers Paper 2

1 a

NICE heart failure guidelines 2003 recommend that all patients with heart failure due to left ventricular dysfunction should be treated with a diuretic and an Angiotensin Converting Enzyme inhibitor (ACEI) or angiotensin II receptor blocker if ACEI is not tolerated. Further treatment options include beta blockers, digoxin and spironolactone. Increasing treatment needs may necessitate specialist input. www.nice.org.uk

2 b

http://www.britishairways.com/travel/healthmedcond/public/en_gb

3 e

Immune thrombocytopenic purpura (ITP) is usually self-limiting in children after a viral illness. Chronic ITP is more common in adults. Antiplatelet autoantibodies cause phagocytic destruction of the platelets. Bleeding, purpura and nose bleeds are common. Retinal and conjunctival haemorrhage is rare. A platelet count of <10 × 10⁹/L, positive anti-platelet IgG autoantibodies and positive antinuclear antibodies in 40% of cases is suggestive of ITP. If symptomatic, or if the platelet count is particularly low, steroids may be used for treatment. Splenectomy may also be required.

4 b

2 months	DTP/IPV/Hib, PCV
3 months	DTP/IPV/Hib, Men C
4 months	DTP/IPV/Hib, Men C, PCV
12 months	Hib/Men C
13 months	MMR, PCV
3 years 4 months to 5 years	dTP/IPV or DTP/IPV, MMR
13–18 years	Td/IPV

D – diphtheria
T – tetanus
P – pertussis
IPV – polio
Hib – Haemophilus influenzae type b
PCV – Pneumococcal conjugate vaccine
MMR – measles mumps and rubella
Refer to www.immunisations.nhs.uk

5 b

The Department of Health will pay practices 95p per patient for producing a plan which sets out how services will be organised for PBC, i.e. DES component 1. More information on PBC can be found on the government website: http://www.dh.gov.uk/en/Policyandguidance/ Organisationpolicy/Commissioning/Practice-basedcommissioning/ index.htm

6 a

Proton pump inhibitors can cause a multitude of mostly gastro-intestinal side-effects.

7 c

Antibiotics are of no benefit in the treatment of uncomplicated acute otitis media. They are, however, recommended: in children under the age of 2 years, if there is a history of recurrent infections and in those who are systemically unwell. Paracetamol may be used for analgesia or as an antipyretic and, if required, amoxicillin is the first-line antibiotic of choice.

8 b

With NSAIDs, pain relief starts after the first dose, the full analgesic effect is achieved after a week and the anti-inflammatory effect can take up to 3 weeks.

9 b

NICE 2007 advises sertraline as the best medical treatment for depression post-MI.

10 j

11 i

12 a

13 d

14 g

15 b

16 k

17 e

18 h

19 f

Arc eye is a common complication in welders or sunbed users who do not use protective glasses. The UV irradiation burns the corneal epithelium causing a painful keratitis. It typically presents with watery eyes and blepharospasm. Treatment includes analgesia, padding the eye and mydriatics if necessary. Spontaneous resolution usually occurs within a day or two.

Herpetic ulcers are particularly worrying to doctors as they can be an iatrogenic complication of ophthalmic steroid use in patients. Ulceration is due to a breach in the epithelial layer which may occur after trauma, for example, in contact-lens wearers. Features include pain, photophobia and blurred vision. Fluroscein drops (orange) stain the ulcer green under blue light. If suspected, specialist ophthalmology input is required for Gram staining and treatment with aciclovir ointment 5 times a day.

Infective conjunctivitis (sticky eye) is very common in children of school/nursery age. This tends to be a self-limiting bacterial or viral infection, which causes a sticky yellow discharge. The eyelids are stuck together and crusty in the morning. The vision tends not to be affected. A Cochrane review concluded that in children, if a week of conservative management is not effective, topical chloramphenicol is a good first-line option. However, pressure from parents usually results in the GP prescribing antibiotics straight away despite guidelines to the contrary.

Subconjunctival haemorrhages are usually of no significant pathology. They can occur after trauma, in hypertensive patients and those who have vomited with some degree of force. It is essential to monitor the blood pressure and any bleeding tendencies if they occur recurrently. No treatment is required for this painless condition.

20 d

Peripheral vascular disease is commonly diagnosed after a patient has noticed intermittent claudication. It tends to be more common in males, smokers and diabetics. Diagnosis can be made on the history using the Edinburgh claudication questionnaire which is 91% specific and 99% sensitive, and measurement of the ankle brachial pressure index (ABPI). Investigations include serum cholesterol and possible angiography.

21 b

Also more common in leukaemia (tissue infiltration).

22 d

90% of specific clinical scenarios as in (d) will be culture positive so the HPA recommends treating without sending an unnecessary urine sample to the lab. Symptoms of UTI include dysuria, frequency, suprapubic tenderness, haematuria, urgency and polyuria. Positive nitrites on dipstick +/– leucocyte +/– protein = likely UTI and also warrant antibiotic treatment.

23 e

According to the BNF: mild = hydrocortisone, moderate = Eumovate®, potent = Betnovate®, very potent = Dermovate®.

24 b

Beta blockers improve survival, reduce hospitalisation due to heart failure (HF), improve symptoms and LV function in patients who have HF due to systolic dysfunction. Contraindications: asthmatics with reversible airways obstruction, reversible limb ischaemia, second- or third-degree heart block, decompensated heart failure. Not all

COPD patients have reversible airways obstruction, therefore can be given beta blockers. The relative risk reduction in mortality is about 35% according to a critical review: McMurray JJ. Major beta blocker mortality trials in chronic heart failure: a critical review. *Heart.* 1999; **82** Suppl 4: IV 14–22. From the BHF fact file *Use of Beta Blockers in Heart Failure*; April 2006 www.bhf.org.uk/factfiles

25 c

Tall stature can be caused by Kleinfelter's syndrome, congenital adrenal hyperplasia, Soto's syndrome and hyperthyroidism.

26 b

Reference: http://guidance.nice.org.uk/CG44. Familiarise yourselves with new NICE guidelines; they are popular exam topics and can afford you easy marks if you have done a bit of reading. It is now good practice to offer the levonorgestrel-releasing intrauterine system as first-line therapy for menorrhagia.

27 b

Also methadone, dihydrocodeine

28 b

Reference: www.resus.org.uk. You must look this up for the current guidelines.

29 c

Reference: http://guidance.nice.org.uk/cg42

30 c

Women are affected twice as often as men ('fat, female, fair, forty, fertile' is the common saying). Obesity, pancreatitis, diabetes, pregnancy and Crohn's increase risk. Ulcerative colitis is associated with bile duct carcinoma.

31 d

Topical metronidazole or topical azelaic acid can be used in the treatment of mild to moderate acne rosacea.

32 c

Incidence Papillary> Follicular> Medullary> Anaplastic> Lymphoma. Age ranges: Papillary 10–40; Follicular 40–60; Anaplastic 50–60. Both medullary and lymphoma at any age.

33 e

NICE Hypertension Guidelines 2006 recommends Step 4 treatment to include further diuretic treatment or alpha-blocker usage or beta blocker usage and consideration of specialist advice. www.nice.org.uk

34 e

Brainstem evoked potentials and otoacoustic emissions are used in the neonatal period and have more than 90% sensitivity for hearing loss of 50 dB or more. The distraction test is no longer so commonly used as it is a tricky test to perform accurately. It is best performed between the ages of 6–9 months. Speech discrimination and threshold audiometry are used mostly in toddlers and older children.

35 c

Reference: Car J. Urinary tract infections in women: diagnosis and management in primary care. *BMJ*. 2006; **332**: 94–7. A clear review article that also has helpful MCQs on UTI management.

36 d

Part C is completed by a registered medical practitioner who is not related in any way to the doctor signing Part B, nor a relative of the patient. Hence, a doctor in another GP surgery is the usual option. This doctor has to have at least 5 years' continuous medical experience.

37 a

Patients should always be advised to gargle with water after usage as oral candidiasis is a potential side-effect. Steroids work over a number of hours and should only be considered for short oral courses. If used in this way they should not cause osteoporosis.

38 a

NICE 2005 Atypical anti-psychotics are used as first-line therapy. www.nice.org.uk

39 a

The policy of immunising susceptible healthcare assistants was introduced in 2003 by the Department of Health after advice from the Joint Committee on Vaccination and Immunisation. The healthcare worker should also be Hepatitis B immune.

40 d

Missed pills can result in ovulation occurring. However, the risk of pregnancy depends on **how many** pills were missed and **when**. Risk is greatest at the beginning or end of a packet when the pill-free interval has been extended. **Ovulation is rare after 7 days of proper pill taking.** Theoretically, the risk of pregnancy is greater if a low-oestrogen pill is being used, i.e. 20mcg. Therefore the Faculty of Family Planning and WHO advise the following:

If one or two 30mcg pills have been missed at any time, or if one 20mcg pill is missed, the woman should take the most recent missed pill as soon as she remembers (she may take two pills together) and continue taking the remaining pills daily at their usual time. She does not require emergency contraception.

If three or more 30mcg pills or two or more 20mcg pills have been missed at any time, she should take the missed pill as soon as she remembers, continue taking the remaining pills daily at the right time and use extra precautions/abstain until she has taken pills for 7 days in a row.

If the pills are missed in week 1, i.e. days 1–7, emergency contraception should be considered if she had unprotected sex in the pill-free interval or in the first week of pill taking. If pills were missed in week 2, i.e. days 8–14, the risk of ovulation is minimal and there is no indication for emergency contraception. If pills were missed in week 3, i.e. days 15–21, she should omit the pill-free interval and start a new pack straight away after finishing the old one. There is no need for emergency contraception as more than 7 pills have been taken in a row in weeks 1 and 2.

Reference: http://www.ffprhc.org.uk/admin/uploads/FirstPresc CombOralContJan06.pdf

41 c

Streptococcus viridans accounts for nearly 50% of infective endocarditis cases and *Staphylococcus aureus* accounts for approximately 20%.

42 e

Smoking status should be recorded for those patients over the age of 15 years. The following website can be used to find the most up to date QOF targets http://www.nhsemployers.org/primary/primary-890.cfm

43 d

The risk of osteoporosis is greatest in thin Caucasian women. The B polymorphism of the Vitamin D receptor gene is over-represented in women with low postmenopausal bone density. Peak bone mass in adulthood is 80% controlled by genetic factors. Exhibiting polymorphism for the Type I collagen gene will increase the risk of osteoporotic fractures. A family history of osteoporosis increases risk. Reference: www.gpnotebook.co.uk

44 c

Both statin therapy and anti-hypertensive therapy, specifically indapamide and perindopril, have been shown to reduce recurrent stroke risk even in patients with normal cholesterol and BP respectively, PROGRESS study and SPARCL study. From the December 2006 edition of the British Heart Foundation factfile, *Early Intervention in Stroke*. Reference: www.bhf.org.uk/factfiles.

45 c

Malaria prophylaxis is not 100% effective at preventing malaria and so should be used in combination with other preventative measures. Patients should be advised to report any illness to a doctor within 1 year of returning from a malaria zone and especially within the first 3 months.

46 b

47 j

48 a

49 g

50 u

51 n

52 r

53 d

Iliotibial band syndrome is described as pain over the outer side of the knee, usually occurring at the middle to end of a run. Treatment includes rest, side stretching, running on softer ground, physiotherapy and correct footwear.

Patello-femoral mal-alignment is a condition in which the patella is not in the correct position in the femoral groove. It leads to non-specific pain around the patella aggravated by prolonged sitting, squatting, going up stairs and running. Treatment includes orthotics to aid pronation, VMO (Vastus medialis obliques) strengthening exercises, physiotherapy and, in severe cases, surgery.

54 d

Manning *et al.* 1978 stated the diagnosis of IBS was based on a link between pain relief and bowel movements, abdominal distension, a sensation of incomplete evacuation, more frequent bowel movements with the onset of pain and also mucus passage. The latest definition is based on the ROME 3 criteria which defines IBS as symptoms of abdominal pain or discomfort for at least three days a month in the past 3 months, together with at least two or more of the following: change in frequency or change in consistency of the stool or pain relieved by defecation. The criteria have to be fulfilled for the past 3 months with the onset of symptoms at least 6 months before diagnosis. Reference: Hayee B, Forgacs I. Psychological approach to managing irritable bowel syndrome. *BMJ*. 2007; **334**: 1105–9.

55 a

On an ECG the QRS complex corresponds with the time taken for the excitation to spread through the ventricles. This is usually less than 0.12 seconds.

56 d

Urethritis is classified as either gonococcal, where *N. gonorrhoea* has been isolated, or non-specific (non-gonococcal), if it has not. NSU can be asymptomatic, but usually presents with urethral discharge/ dysuria. The commonest cause is *Chlamydia trachomatis*, in up to 50% of cases. It is sexually transmitted and contact tracing is part of its management. Recommended treatment is doxycycline 100mg bd for 7 days or azithromycin 1g stat orally. It is diagnosed by demonstrating the presence of more than a certain amount of pus cells from the anterior urethra on microscopy. Reference: http://www.bashh.org/ guidelines

57 b

Seborrhoeic dermatitis is thought to be caused by a fungal infection.

58 e

Subclinical hypothyroidism should be confirmed by repeating thyroid function tests 3 months after the first raised TSH level is noted. Treatment is recommended but may be deferred if the TSH is only slightly raised, i.e. less than 10mU/L, and antithyroid antibodies test negative. The annual rate of progression for women with subclinical hypothyroidism to clinical hypothyroidism is approximately 4.3% if antibodies are present, and 2.6 % if the antibodies are not present. Progression in men is more likely.

59 c

Multiple myeloma is a malignant neoplasm of plasma cells that can cause pathological fractures. Diagnosis is confirmed by serum electrophoresis and Bence-Jones proteinuria.

60 e

The Committee on the Safety of Medicines advice states that bupropion is contraindicated in patients with a history of seizures, eating disorders and bipolar disorder. It is to be prescribed with caution when patients are on medication that lower the seizure threshold, e.g. antimalarials and antidepressants, and used only when the benefits outweigh the risks.

61 b

Down's syndrome (Trisomy 21) sufferers display typical facies, e.g. eyes that slant upwards with prominent epicanthic folds, a flat occiput, a flat bridge of the nose, abundant neck skin and dysplastic ears. Other features include a protruding tongue, single palmer crease, incurved fifth finger and Brushfield spots in the iris. Associated medical problems include learning difficulties and Alzheimer's dementia, hypothyroidism, congenital heart defects such as atrial/ventricular septal defects, and gastrointestinal congenital malformations such as duodenal atresia.

62 d

63 k

64 b

65 f

66 n

67 c

To help you answer any question such as this, memorise the following table and definitions. It takes no time to construct a table in the exam with the information given and you can be sure of an accurate answer every time.

	Disease positive	Disease negative	Total
Test positive	True positive = a	False positive = b	a+b
Test negative	False negative = c	True negative = d	c+d
	a+c	b+d	a+b+c+d

	Bowel cancer	No bowel cancer	Total
FOB positive	290	100	390
FOB negative	110	500	610
	400	600	1000

PPV = the ability of a screening test to predict the disease-positive people in those with a positive result. PPV = a/a+b = 290/390 = 74%

NPV = the ability of a screening test to predict the disease-negative people in those with a negative result. NPV= d/c+d = 500/610 = 82%

Sensitivity = the true positive rate; i.e. the proportion of people with a positive result who do have the disease. Sensitivity = a/a+c = 290/400 = 72.5%

Specificity = the true negative rate; i.e. the proportion of people with a negative result who do not have the disease. Specificity = d/b+d = 500/600 = 83%

Number of false positive results = 100

Number of false negative results = 110

68 b

Mitral stenosis is usually caused by rheumatic heart disease. Symptoms include dyspnoea, palpitations, haemoptysis and right heart failure. Signs include: a malar flush which may be a sign of peripheral cyanosis; a left parasternal heave, and an undisplaced tapping apex beat. The pulse is of normal character. After an opening snap there is a loud S1 heart sound. A mid-diastolic murmur best heard at the apex is classical. Chest x-ray and echocardiogram are essential investigations. Diuretics and digoxin may be useful treatment options but mitral valve replacement may be necessary. Endocarditis prophylactic antibiotics are required.

69 a

Clinical features include vulnerability to infections, anaemia, bleeding and easy bruising. AML classically leads to leukaemic cell deposition in the gums, causing hypertrophy.

70 a

Measles is an RNA virus with an incubation period of 8–12 days. Prodromal symptoms include cough, coryza and conjunctivitis. White spots on the buccal mucosa (Koplik's spots), otitis media and a rash that starts behind the ears are classic features. Serious complications include pneumonia, encephalitis and deafness. Roseola infantum (a DNA herpes virus) tends to affect younger children and the rash classically appears around the neck, trunk and face as the fever subsides. Serious complications such as meningitis and encephalitis may arise.

71 b

It is essential to rule out biliary atresia if jaundice is present at 14 days and the child is not thriving. It tends to be more common in boys. It is found in 1 in 15 000 live births. Hepatosplenomegaly may be present. Investigations may include CT or nuclear medicine scanning and treatment is surgical.

72 a

Phaeochromocytoma is a noradrenaline-secreting tumour of the adrenal glands with a peak incidence in the 30- to 40-year age group. Acute symptoms include tachycardia, anxiety, sweating and headaches. Hypertension which is unresponsive to medication is the usual presenting feature.

73 e

The gene for sickle-cell anaemia follows an autosomal recessive inheritance pattern.

74 c

ASCOT looked at amlodipine and perindopril versus beta blocker and diuretics in reducing the risk of coronary events, new-onset diabetes, stroke and mortality. Due to obvious benefits, the trial was stopped early by the Data Safety Monitoring Board – finishing in 2004. It involved more than 19 000 patients with hypertension and at least three other risk factors. The amlodipine/perindopril combination showed a decrease in new-onset diabetes of 30%, in cardiovascular disease of 24% and in death by any cause of 11%. The lipid-lowering arm of the trial comprised 10 305 patients with non-fasting total cholesterol levels of 6.5mmol/L or less, who were randomised to additional treatment with atorvastatin (10mg daily) or placebo. Sever PS *et al.* Prevention of coronary and stroke events with atorvastatin in hypertensive patients who have average or lower-than-average cholesterol concentrations, in the Anglo-Scandinavian Cardiac Outcomes Trial Lipid-Lowering Arm (ASCOT-LLA): a multicentre randomised trial. *Lancet.* 2003; **361**: 1149–58.

75 a

76 b

Temporal arteritis is treated with oral prednisolone at a dose between 40 and 60mg. However, if there is loss of vision, intravenous steroids are used.

77 e

78 q

79 f

80 g

81 o

It only takes a few minutes to learn this and again, you stand to gain easy marks for a potentially difficult question.

82 e

The foods listed are all sources of oxalate except oranges. Calcium oxalate is a type of renal stone. Immobilisation, dehydration, anatomical anomalies, gout, hyperparathyroidism, diuretics and anticonvulsants can all increase the risk of renal stones.

83 e

HCV antibodies can take up to 3 months to become positive. NICE 2006 states treatment should be with Interferon alpha and Ribavirin for mild chronic hepatitis. In 1991 blood products in the UK began to be screened for HCV. Only 20% of people infected will develop acute hepatitis and the greatest risk of transmission in the UK is from intravenous drug use.

84 b

Permethrin 5% needs to be applied over the whole body and left for 8–12 hours before it is washed off. Malathion should be applied for 24 hours. Both are re-applied after a week. The whole household should be treated. The itch may benefit from a sedating antihistamine, e.g. chlorphenamine.

85 d

Vitamin D deficiency, Ricket's disease, is common in babies fed solely on milk until age 18 months. It is uncommon these days. It is commoner in Afro-Caribbean or Asian children. The child may display bowed legs, splaying of the wrists and ankles and may have a 'rickety rosary' (the enlargement of the costochondral joints) of the rib cage. Vitamin A deficiency can lead to blindness. Vitamin B deficiency can cause lethargy, paraesthesiae and heart palpitations. Vitamin C deficiency (scurvy) can cause bleeding gums and mucus membranes, joint pain and swelling. Vitamin E deficiency causes neurological symptoms and haemolytic anaemia.

86 c

According to NICE guidelines, it is recommended that a statin for primary prevention be started at a level of 20% 10-year cardiovascular risk. www.nice.org.uk

87 b

Doxycycline is contraindicated. Recommended treatment by BASHH is erythromycin 500mg qds for 7 days OR erythromycin 500mg bd for 14 days OR amoxicillin 500mg tds for 7 days OR azithromycin 1g stat po – this may be less effective though. Remember contact tracing. Transmission to the neonate may result in neonatal conjunctivitis or pneumonia. http://www.bashh.org/guidelines

88 e

Osteoporosis is also associated with steroid use, premature menopause, amenorrhoea, Turner's syndrome, hyperthyroidism and heparin.

89 d

This is erysipelas, most commonly caused by *Streptococcus* or *Staphylococcus* species. Therefore the treatment of choice is Phenoxymethylpenicillin.

90 a

Coronary artery bypass grafting (CABG) is an option if medical management fails or if there is left main stem disease. It can also be used as alternative to failed angioplasty. The patient's own saphenous vein and internal mammary artery may be used. In the case of the latter, chest wall numbness can be a problem. Clopidogrel is used routinely after operations. Patients are allowed to drive 1 month after surgery.

91 b

Gestational hypertension is a BP of >140/90mmHg, detected after 20 weeks' gestation in the absence of proteinuria and resolves spontaneously within 3 months of delivery.

92 d

93 f

94 a

95 b

96 h

97 j

Asthma is a common childhood disease which presents as a night-time cough in a well child or as exercise induced cough/wheeze/shortness of breath. Diagnosis is made by peak flow variability or bronchodilator responsiveness.

Bronchial carcinoma is the commonest cancer in the UK and is the third most common cause of death in the UK. Bronchial carcinoma can present with non-specific symptoms and signs, e.g. cough, weight loss or general malaise. Chest pain, haemoptysis or a hoarse voice may be more indicative of serious lung pathology.

Pancoast's syndrome is an apical tumour which infiltrates the sympathetic chain causing an ipsilateral Horner's syndrome. It spreads to the brachial plexus causing wasting of the small muscles of the hand, and laryngeal nerve palsy causes a hoarse voice.

Pulmonary embolus is fatal in 1 in 10 cases. Risk factors include: contraceptive pill usage; immobility; smoking; malignancy; pregnancy, and past history. Presentation includes pleuritic chest pain, dyspnoea and haemoptysis. Chest x-ray, D-dimer and CT Pulmonary Angiography may all be necessary for diagnosis.

A spontaneous pneumothorax must be considered in a tall thin man with sudden onset of pleuritic chest pain, dyspnoea or syncope as a pleural bleb ruptures. In patients over the age of 40 years, chronic obstructive pulmonary disease is the usual underlying cause. Chest x-ray is required for diagnosis and, if small, the pneumothorax can spontaneously resolve.

Atypical pneumonia can be caused by *Chlamydia*, *Mycoplasma* and *Legionella* species. An atypical pathogen should be considered if symptoms are slow to resolve. They are more common in immuno-compromised patients. Usual symptoms include a persistent dry cough, anorexia and weight loss. Chest x-ray usually shows patchy consolidation.

Legionella pneumophila must be considered in patients who have recently travelled abroad as the pathogen tends to breed in warm stagnant water such as is found in air conditioning systems. The patient may present with extra-pulmonary signs initially such as diarrhoea, vomiting, confusion and delirium. The patient may be very unwell. Diagnosis is with serology and treatment with erythromycin is effective.

98 c

HIV-positive patients can receive MMR vaccine unless severely immunocompromised; however, they should not be immunised with BCG or yellow fever. Rabies is an inactivated virus.

99 a

This is an unlicensed indication, however there is no substitute for prior acclimatisation. www.bnf.org

100 d

The NHS Bowel Cancer Screening Programme began in April 2006 and is being rolled out over the next 3 years. Screening tests will be sent to everyone aged between 60–69 years although those over 70 can request a test for themselves. GPs are not directly involved. The faecal occult blood (FOB) test is to be used for screening, with participants expected to put a faecal sample on a card and send it back to the lab. Results will be available in 2 weeks. Ninety-eight per cent of participants will be expected to have a negative result and up to 4% will require re-testing due to unclear results. Around 2% are expected to have a positive result and require further investigation. There are five screening hubs that will receive tests from designated areas of the country. The pilot screening programme evaluation has shown the uptake to be around 50% for FOB tests. Reference: www.cancerscreening.nhs.uk/bowel

Paper 3

1 Aspirin is known to be beneficial in cardiovascular disease. What one other condition has been shown in observational studies to benefit from aspirin?

  a Alzheimer's disease

  b Irritable bowel disease

  c Parkinson's disease

  d Asthma

  e Thyroid dysfunction

2 What is the normal PR interval shown in an ECG?

  a 0.5–0.62s

  b 0.12–0.2s

  c 0.2–0.32s

  d 0.05–0.12s

  e 0.25–0.35s

3 A 3-year-old child presents with malaise and recurrent infections. Her mother states that she bruises easily. On examination, she is pale, widespread bruises of different ages are seen and hepato-splenomegaly is palpable. What is the most likely diagnosis?

  a Scurvy

  b Acute leukaemia

  c Henoch Schonlein Purpura

  d Non-accidental injury

  e Normal

4   Which one of the following is not true about estimated glomerular filtration rate (eGFR)?

a   eGFR is an estimate.

b   eGFR needs extra calculations for different races.

c   Creatinine levels must be stable over the time the eGFR is calculated.

d   eGFR is not valid for those under 18 years of age.

e   eGFR is the most accurate near the normal value.

5   Which one of the following statements is not true about genital herpes?

a   Genital herpes can be acquired from contact with lesions from non-mucosal surfaces.

b   Typing of the infection is useful in managing recurrent genital herpes.

c   Typing of the infection is useful in the initial attack.

d   Antivirals do not eradicate the infection or latent virus.

e   Aciclovir, valaciclovir and famciclovir all decrease the severity and duration of the clinical episode.

6   Which one of the following is not true about economic analysis?

a   It involves the use of analysis to define choices in resource allocation.

b   It takes into account direct, indirect and intangible costs.

c   Cost/benefit analysis measures the outcome in monetary units.

d   Cost-utility analysis measures outcomes in monetary units.

e   Cost-effectiveness analysis compares expenditure with outcome.

7 Which one of the following is not true regarding the risk of developing deep vein thrombosis (DVT)?

a DVT occurs in over 40% of patients having major orthopaedic surgery.

b A body mass index (BMI) over 30 is a risk factor for developing DVT.

c Risk factors include immobility associated with continuous travel of more than 1 hour's duration in the month before surgery.

d Patients should be advised to stop taking the oral contraceptive pill 4 weeks prior to elective surgery.

e If patients have more than one risk factor for developing DVT they require prophylaxis with low molecular weight heparin when undergoing surgery.

8 Symbicort® is a combination of which of the following asthma drugs?

a Budesonide and formoterol

b Fluticasone and salmeterol

c Budesonide and sodium cromoglicate

d Beclomethasone and formoterol

e Ipratroprium and salmeterol

9 A 65-year-old gentleman presents with new onset epigastric pain. He has been a smoker for 50 years. He has also become increasingly breathless on exertion. On examination you note he has cracks on the side of his mouth. What would be your choice for further management?

a Chest x-ray

b Urgently refer for oesophogastroduodenoscopy (OGD)

c Treat with ferrous sulphate

d Trial of a proton pump inhibitor

e *Helicobacter pylori* serology

10 A 28-year-old woman presents with tiredness and weight loss over the past 6 months. On examination you notice she has dark pigmentation in her palmar creases. Blood test results are as follows:

Sodium	122mmol/L	(133–147mmol/L)
Potassium	5.8mmol/L	(3.5–5.0mmol/L)
Albumin	58g/L	(35–50g/L)
Urea	9mmol/L	(2.5–7.5mmol/L)

Which one of the following is the most likely diagnosis?

a Cushing's syndrome

b Conn's syndrome

c Addison's disease

d Pheochromocytoma

e Diabetes insipidus

Using the list of values given answer the following questions (Questions 11 to 14). Options may be used once, more than once or not at all.

List of values: 2, 3, 30, 9, 15, 20, 20, 20, 61, 72, 47, 99, 99, 103, 105

Options:

a 103

b 3

c 15

d 20

e 72

f 99

g 105

h 61

i 47

j 2

k 105

l 30

11 Which number represents the mode in the list of values?

12 Which number represents the mean in the list of values?

13 Which number represents the median in the list of values?

14 Which number represents the range in the list of values?

15 Which one of the following statements is true regarding osteoporosis?

   a 35% of women aged 75–85 years have severe osteoporosis.

   b About one-third of Caucasian women will have at least one osteoporotic vertebral fracture by the age of 70 years.

   c The incidence of osteoporosis is higher in Afro Caribbeans.

   d About one-third of women aged 90 years will have had a hip fracture.

   e The incidence of femoral neck fracture increases markedly after the age of 60 years, more so in women than in men, and more so in Caucasians than in other races.

16 Concerning environmental and personal hygiene measures in the treatment of threadworm (*Enterobias vermicularis*), which one of the following statements is correct?

   a Environmental and personal hygiene measures are of no proven benefit.

   b There is no need to use separate towels.

   c The eggs are not infectious once they are removed from the body.

   d Fingernails should be kept short.

   e Advise patients to wear loose-fitting underwear at night.

17 Which one of the following statements is true about aortic stenosis (AS)?

   a Can be caused by hyperthyroidism.

   b Usually causes sudden death.

   c Is associated with a slow rising pulse.

   d Causes a displaced apex.

   e ECG shows large P-waves.

18 Side-effects of tetracycline include all of the following except which one?

a Oesophageal irritation

b Impotence

c Nausea and vomiting

d Photosensitivity rash

e Diarrhoea

19 Concerning yellow fever vaccination, which one of the following statements is true?

a All travellers to India should be vaccinated.

b Revaxis® is a trade name.

c The vaccine is inactivated.

d It can be given safely to pregnant women.

e Immunity takes 10 days to develop after vaccination.

20 At what age would you expect a baby to be able to smile responsively?

a 4 weeks

b 8 weeks

c 6 weeks

d 2 weeks

e 10 weeks

21 A 40-year-old smoker complains of a 5-week history of cough with white phlegm. On examination, he is afebrile and the chest is clear. What would be your first course of action?

a Review in 2 weeks.

b Prescribe amoxicillin 500mg tds.

c Prescribe a trial of an inhaler.

d Organise a walk-in chest x-ray.

e Refer to routine respiratory clinic.

22 Under the new Department of Health guidelines, who is not offered annual influenza vaccination routinely?

a Carer to a patient >70 years

b Patients aged over 65 years

c Patients with diabetes

d Patients with asthma

e Patients with cystic fibrosis

23 According to the 2007 British Association for the Study of Headache (BASH) guidelines on treating migraine, which of the following drugs has no place in treating an acute attack?

a Paracetamol

b Metoclopramide

c Codeine phosphate

d Sumatriptan

e Rectal Diclofenac

24 What is a recognised treatment for chlamydia from the following options?

a Erythromycin 500mg bd for 14 days

b Ciprofloxacin 500mg stat dose

c Cefixime 400mg stat dose

d Doxycycline 400mg tds for 7 days

e Azithromycin 200mg bd for 3 days

Choose the most likely diagnosis from the list below for each clinical scenario (Questions 25 to 30). Options may be used once, more than once or not at all.

a Breast carcinoma

b Breast cyst

c Fibroadenoma

d Breast abscess

e Fat necrosis

f Lipoma

g Galactocoele

h Duct ectasia

i Fibroadenosis/Cyclical mastalgia

j Intraductal papilloma

25 A 30-year-old woman presents with pre-menstrual breast pain and a small amount of green nipple discharge at times. On examination, thickened breast tissue in the upper, outer quadrants is palpable bilaterally. No lymphadenopathy is present.

26 A 20-year-old woman presents with a 4-week history of a single breast lump. On examination, a smooth, firm, mobile lump is palpable in the left breast.

27 A 55-year-old woman presents with painful breasts bilaterally. She has noted some thick creamy nipple discharge. On examination, the subareolar regions are erythematous and there is no lymphadenopathy.

28 A 30-year-old woman presents with a painful breast lump after being hit in the chest with a tennis ball. On examination an irregular, hard lump tethered to the skin is palpable.

29 A breast-feeding mother presents with a painful and swollen right breast. On examination, she is pyrexial and the breast is enlarged, red and tender. No discrete lump is palpable.

30 A 54-year-old woman presents with a breast lump found on self-examination. A tender, discrete craggy lump is palpable. A small amount of bloody nipple discharge is seen.

31 According to the February 2007 Department of Health White Paper, *Trust, Assurance and Safety: the regulation of health professionals in the 21st century*, which of the following statements is true?

   a All doctors will hold a licence to practise which will enable them to remain on the medical register and which must be renewed every 2 years.

   b Specialist recertification will apply to all specialists, excluding general practitioners.

   c The appraisal process will include 'summative' elements that confirm a doctor has objectively met the standards expected, e.g. an applied knowledge test.

d Only doctors who work in the NHS will be expected to go through the process of revalidation.

e The appraisal process will lose its 'formative' components.

32 According to the NICE Hypertension guidelines 2006 what is the most appropriate treatment for a 45-year-old Caucasian male with a sustained blood pressure of >170/100mmHg?

a Ramipril

b Atenolol

c Losartan

d Amlodipine

e Propranolol

33 Which of the following conditions does not have approval from the Advisory Committee on Borderline Substances (ACBS) to have food products prescribed on a FP10?

a Crohn's disease

b Phenylketonuria

c Lactose intolerance

d Vomiting in infancy

e Irritable Bowel Syndrome (IBS)

34 Regarding the treatment of depression, which one of the following statements is true?

a Selective serotonin reuptake inhibitors (SSRIs) should be prescribed to all patients with depression.

b Self-help books have no place in treatment options and can only lead to patients feeling helpless and worthless.

c St John's wart has been proven to be no better than placebo.

d Cognitive behavioural therapy (CBT) is of no use.

e An assessment of the suicide risk should be carried out on each patient.

35 What is the pattern of inheritance of infantile polycystic renal disease?

  a Autosomal dominant

  b Autosomal recessive

  c X-linked recessive

  d X-linked dominant

  e Multifactorial

36 Which one of the following is not a known side-effect of steroids?

  a Peptic ulcer formation

  b Hypothyroidism

  c Psychosis

  d Osteoporosis

  e Pancreatitis

37 A 60-year-old male suddenly loses his vision. On examination, the retina appears white with a cherry-red spot at the macula. What is the diagnosis?

  a Occlusion of the central retinal artery

  b Occlusion of the central retinal vein

  c Vitreous haemorrhage

  d Retinal detachment

  e Branch occlusion of central retinal vein

38 Which of following is defined as a detailed review of similar studies that meet strict criteria?

  a Cohort study

  b Retrospective study

  c Meta-analysis

  d Systematic review

  e Qualitative analysis

39 Which one of the following statements regarding pregnancy and maternity leave is not true?

a Employees can take maternity leave any time after 29 weeks' gestation.

b Two weeks' maternity leave is compulsory after the baby's birth.

c A due date after 1 April 2007 entitles an employee to 52 weeks' maternity leave.

d Pension contributions continue to be paid by the employer during the period of paid maternity leave.

e Full maternity leave entitlement prevails in the event of a stillbirth at 22 weeks' gestation.

40 When administering basic life support, what is the optimal depth for chest compressions according to the current UK Resuscitation Council Guidelines?

a 1–2cm

b 2–3cm

c 3–4cm

d 4–5cm

e 5–6cm

41 What is the false positive rate for Prostate Specific Antigen to detect prostate cancer?

a Approximately 40%

b Approximately 55%

c Approximately 66%

d Approximately 26%

e Approximately 87%

42 Which one of the following statements is not true about tuberculosis (TB)?

a A Mantoux test may be falsely negative in patients with HIV.

b Previous BCG vaccination prevents HIV-positive patients contracting TB.

c Colour vision needs to be tested prior to TB treatment.

d There is a increased rate of reactivation of latent TB in HIV-positive patients.

e Acid-fast bacilli may be found in the sputum.

43 A 12-year-old girl presents to the GP with short stature. On examination she has a wide carrying angle and a webbed neck. Which syndrome is most likely?

a Down's syndrome

b Turner's syndrome

c Kleinfelter's syndrome

d Fragile X syndrome

e Edward's syndrome

Select the appropriate time interval after which airlines and the World Health Organisation will allow someone to fly with the clinical conditions listed below (in Questions 44 to 51). Each option may be used once, more than once or not at all.

a 6 months

b 48 hours

c 2 weeks

d 1 year

e 7 days

f 3 months

g 10 days

h 3 weeks

i 4 weeks

j 2 months

k 24 hours

44 Simple fracture with no plaster cast

45 Minimum age of child before first flight

46 Myocardial infarction

47 Haemorrhagic stroke

48 Eye surgery

49 Grand mal seizure

50 Plaster cast applied to fracture

51 Pneumothorax

52 What is the starting dose of methotrexate in rheumatoid arthritis?
  a 2.5mg daily
  b 5mg weekly
  c 7.5mg weekly
  d 5mg alternate days
  e 5mg daily

53 A 26-year-old male presents with a verruca on his foot. Which one of the following statements is true of cryotherapy?
  a Cryotherapy is not painful.
  b Cryotherapy may result in permanent hypopigmentation of the skin.
  c Cryotherapy successfully cures warts after two treatments in 70% of cases.
  d Cryotherapy is the only option for wart removal.
  e Cryotherapy has been shown to be more effective than salicylic acid paint.

54 What size needle is recommended by the Chief Medical Officer to administer the Pneumococcal vaccine?

a 21 gauge (green)

b 23 gauge (blue)

c 25 gauge (orange)

d 18 gauge (pink)

e 20 gauge (yellow)

55 What is the chance of producing a child with cystic fibrosis (CF) from a non-consanguineous couple of European descent?

a 1 in 250

b 1 in100

c 1 in 25

d 1 in 2500

e 1 in 1000

56 According to the International Diabetes Federation, metabolic syndrome is diagnosed if a man has a waist circumference of >94cm and two of four other criteria. Which of the following is not one of the four criteria?

a A high-density lipoprotein (HDL) level <1.0mmol/L

b A total cholesterol level >5mmol/L

c A blood pressure reading of >130/85 mmHg

d A triglyceride level >1.7mmol/L

e A fasting plasma glucose level >5.6mmol/L

57 A patient presents with a swollen painful right ankle. Which one of the following clinical features would indicate the need for an x-ray?

a Pain over the anterior edge of the lateral malleolus

b Ability to weight bear initially but difficulty increased after 2 hours

c Pain over the anterior edge of the medial malleolus

d Pain over the base of the 5th metatarsal

e Extreme swelling and bruising

58 Sequelae of genital *Chlamydia* infection include all of the following except:

a Perihepatitis

b Conjunctivitis

c Cervical cancer

d Infertility

e Arthritis

59 According to the World Health Organisation (WHO), which of the following is a criterion to make a diagnosis of diabetes mellitus?

a A random plasma glucose level of 10.4mmol/L

b A fasting plasma glucose level of 7.4mmol/L

c Detecting +++ glycosuria on urine dipstick

d A capillary blood glucose level of 4.8mmol/L

e A 2-hour, post 75g glucose load, plasma glucose level of 8.7mmol/L

60 A diagnosis of chronic obstructive pulmonary disease (COPD) can be made if FEV1/FVC <0.7 (i.e. <70%) and if the FEV1 is:

a <70% predicted

b >70% predicted

c <75% predicted

d <80% predicted

e >80% predicted

61 Which one of the following does not increase the risk of gastro-intestinal bleeding?

a Diclofenac

b Paroxetine

c Amytriptylline

d Prednisolone

e Aspirin

62 You are called to a 75-year-old patient's house by a concerned neighbour. The patient lives alone and has no social support. You notice she is very thin and has peri-follicular haemorrhages on her lower limbs. On further questioning, she complains of spontaneous bleeding of the gums. What is her diagnosis?

    a Vitamin C deficiency

    b Vitamin B12 deficiency

    c Vitamin A deficiency

    d Folate deficiency

    e Vitamin K deficiency

63 What colour is a Med 3 form?

    a White

    b Pink

    c Green

    d Yellow

    e Blue

64 According to the June 2006 NICE guidelines for the treatment of atrial fibrillation (AF), which statement is not true?

    a Rhythm control should be attempted first for patients over the age of 65 who have persistent AF.

    b Rate control should be attempted first for patients over the age of 65 who have persistent AF.

    c Rhythm control should be attempted first for patients with persistent AF who are symptomatic.

    d Rhythm control should be attempted first for patients who present with lone AF for the first time.

    e If AF persists despite a corrected cause or precipitant, rhythm control should be attempted first.

65 A recommended treatment for uncomplicated anogenital *Neisseria gonorrhoea* infection is:

    a Cefixime 400mg po stat

    b Ciprofloxacin 250mg po stat

    c Amoxicillin 1g po stat

d Phenoxymethylpenicillin 250mg po stat

e Erythromycin 500mg bd for 5 days

Match the most likely diagnosis to the clinical scenarios described below (in Questions 66 to 70). Each option may be used once, more than once or not at all.

a Pyloric stenosis

b Epididymo-orchitis

c Acute abdominal obstruction

d Urinary tract infection

e Intussusception

f Testicular torsion

g Physiological abdominal pain

h Constipation

i Gastrointestinal infection

j Overfeeding

k Hirschprung's disease

66 A mother brings her 7-week-old boy to the accident and emergency department. She reports he vomits after every feed. On further questioning, she reports feeding him 150mls every 2 hours. On examination, he is afebrile with a soft abdomen. He is of normal weight.

67 A 15-year-old boy presents complaining of a sore throat and a 3-day history of lower abdominal pain and fever. On examination, he has a tender, erythematous, enlarged right testicle.

68 A 1-year-old boy presents with colicky abdominal pain, drawing up his legs in distress. Earlier he had been vomiting. He begins to pass loose stools containing mucus. On examination, he has an abdominal mass.

69 A hungry 6-week-old boy presents with vomiting after every feed. He is usually constipated. On examination, his weight and length are below the 25th centile.

70 A 15-year-old boy presents to the accident and emergency department with a 1-day history of right iliac fossa pain and vomiting. On examination, he has a swollen, hard, red right testicle.

71 According to the Health Protection Agency, what is a recommended first-line treatment for uncomplicated urinary tract infection?

   a Trimethoprim 200mg bd for 5 days

   b Nitrofurantoin 50mg qds for 6 days

   c Trimethoprim 200mg bd for 7 days

   d Amoxicillin 500mg tds for 7 days

   e Nitrofurantoin 100mg qds for 3 days

72 Which one of the following statements is true of the drug finasteride?

   a It is licensed for all types of baldness.

   b It is licensed for females with male pattern baldness.

   c Side-effects include gynaecomastia.

   d It increases the prostate-specific antigen (PSA) level.

   e It has no effect on the prostate.

73 Regarding delays in treatment for acute myocardial infarction (MI), which one of the following statements is not true, according to the British Heart Foundation?

   a Around 30% of people who die of an acute MI do so before reaching hospital.

   b Mortality from an acute MI is twice as high in patients treated 4–6 hours after the onset of symptoms as it is in those treated within 1–2 hours.

   c Although medical services are getting better at minimising delays to treatment, a major cause of delay is the failure of chest-pain victims to call for help.

   d People with a past history of ischaemic heart disease tend to call for help earlier if experiencing chest pain.

e The British Heart Foundation (BHF) launched a national public awareness campaign, 'Doubt Kills', in 2006 to advise people to call for help early if experiencing chest pain.

74 The ESPRIT trial in 2006 compared which therapies to reduce the risk of recurrent ischaemic stroke?

a Aspirin vs clopidogrel

b Aspirin vs warfarin

c Aspirin vs dipyridamole

d Aspirin vs aspirin+dipyridamole

e Aspirin vs aspirin+clopidogrel

75 Concerning patients who have had a splenectomy, which one of the following statements is true?

a Life-long prophylaxis with ciprofloxacin is required.

b *Haemophilus influenzae* type b immunisation is not recommended.

c Mortality rates from infection are highest in the first 2 years after splenectomy.

d Febrile illnesses can be managed by a 'watch and wait' attitude.

e Splenectomy is not a criterion for a medical alert bracelet.

76 A 16-year-old girl presents with an itchy red patch around her umbilicus and you diagnose nickel allergy. What type of hypersensitivity reaction is this?

a I

b II

c III

d IV

e V

77 With respect to the NICE 2005 guidance on the secondary prevention of osteoporotic fragility fractures in postmenopausal women, which one of the following groups should not be on oral bisphosphonate treatment?

  a Women over 75 years without DEXA scanning.

  b Women with a body mass index (BMI) <19kg/m² without DEXA scanning.

  c Women aged 65–74 years and DEXA scan confirms osteoporosis.

  d Women with a family history of maternal hip fracture before age 75 years and DEXA scan confirms osteoporosis.

  e Women with rheumatoid arthritis and DEXA scan confirms osteoporosis.

78 A 28-year-old lady with a body mass index (BMI) of 38, who has not travelled abroad recently, is not on regular medication and has an alcohol intake of 20 units per week has some routine blood tests performed which show the following. What is the diagnosis?

Full blood count	Normal	
Bilirubin	4µmol/L	(0–20µmol/L)
Alkaline phosphatase (ALP)	67IU/L	(35–104IU/L)
Aspartate transaminase (AST)	38IU/L	(<31IU/L)
Alanine transaminase (ALT)	69IU/L	(<31IU/L)
Gamma gluteryl transferase (GGT)	43IU/L	(5–36IU/L)

  a Hypothyroidism

  b Alcoholic liver disease

  c Viral hepatitis

  d Fatty liver infiltration

  e Hepatoma

79 Which one of the following statements is true of Gardasil® vaccine?

  a It is effective against all types of herpes virus.

  b It is administered as a one-off dose.

  c It can prevent all types of cervical cancer.

d It should be given to girls before they become sexually active.

e It is administered subcutaneously.

80 Concerning head lice, select one correct answer.

a Affected children should be excluded from school.

b Malathion treatment is superior to 'wet combing'.

c Most commonly affects children from 6 months to 3 years.

d Resistance has developed to some insecticides.

e Shampoos are the most effective form of treatment.

Match the following clinical scenarios with one of the diagnoses listed below (in Questions 81 to 86). Each diagnosis may be used once, more than once, or not at all.

a Ectopic pregnancy

b Threatened miscarriage

c Inevitable miscarriage

d Missed miscarriage

e Septic miscarriage

f Placental abruption

g Uterine rupture

h Placenta praevia

i Placenta accraeta

j Hyperemesis gravidarum

k Abnormal lie

l Fibroid uterus

m Appendicitis

n Pyelonephritis

o Multiple pregnancy

p Hydatidiform molar pregnancy

81 A 24-year-old woman presents with 8 weeks' amenorrhea. She complains of spotting vaginally. She has no abdominal pain. When examined her cervical os is closed. Her uterus size is of 6 weeks' gestation.

82 A 36-year-old woman is 23 weeks pregnant and admits to being a smoker. She complains of crampy abdominal pains and reduced fetal movements. There is no vaginal bleeding. On examination she is tachycardic and her uterus feels firm.

83 A 34-year-old woman is 12 weeks pregnant and presents with severe nausea, vomiting and vaginal bleeding. Blood pressure is 149/95mmHg. Her uterus size is 16 weeks' gestation. No fetal heart is heard.

84 A 28-year-old woman presents with severe right-sided iliac fossa pain associated with nausea. She took the emergency contraceptive pill 7 weeks ago and has not seen her period. On examination she is tachycardic. She is not bleeding vaginally.

85 A 33-year-old woman in her second pregnancy presents at 34 weeks with pain in her abdomen and reduced fetal movements. You notice a tender Caesarean section scar and no fetal heart. She is tachycardic and hypotensive.

86 A 19-year-old woman who is 9 weeks pregnant, presents with fever, vomiting and severe right-sided abdominal pain. She was blindly treated for cystitis one week previously.

87 Malarone® is a combination of which two drugs?
   a Atovaquone and proguanil
   b It is not a combination medication.
   c Mefloquine and proguanil
   d Doxycycline and chloroquine
   e Proguanil and chloroquine

88 Concerning temporomandibular joint dysfunction (TMJD) which one of the following is not true?
   a Approximately one-third of people will suffer from TMJD in their lifetime.
   b It tends to be worse in the morning.
   c Normal jaw opening is limited.
   d Erythrocyte sedimentation rate (ESR) should be checked.

e Selective serotonin re-uptake inhibitors are a useful treatment option.

89 Concerning blepharitis, which one of the following is true?
   a Topical chloramphenicol is the treatment of choice.
   b Eyelid hygiene is first-line treatment.
   c It is an acute painful condition.
   d Contact lenses may not be worn.
   e Visual acuity is impaired.

90 What is the most common cause of death in children in England and Wales?
   a Fire
   b Drowning
   c Falls
   d Poisoning
   e Road traffic accidents

91 Which part of the cremation form pertains to the cremation of body parts retained for medico-legal and other purposes?
   a A
   b B
   c C
   d F
   e FF

92 According to NICE guidance, which of the following is not true about beta blockers?
   a The dose should be doubled every week.
   b Aim for the target dose or highest level tolerated.
   c Check blood electrolytes and renal function 2 weeks after initiating treatment.
   d Check blood tests 2 weeks after the final dose increase.
   e Titrate the dose down where necessary.

93 Which one statement is not true about acute lymphoblastic leukaemia (ALL)?

    a White blood cell count >50 × 10^9/L is associated with a worse prognosis.

    b Female gender is associated with a worse prognosis.

    c Bulky organomegaly is associated with a worse prognosis.

    d Central nervous disease is associated with a worse prognosis.

    e Bulky lymphadenopathy is associated with a worse prognosis.

94 The drug of choice for the treatment of depression in patients over the age of 60 years is:

    a Imipramine

    b Paroxetine

    c Duloxetine

    d Haloperidol

    e Venlaflaxine

95 Which one of the following statements is true concerning tonsillitis?

    a Antibiotics are needed in all cases.

    b Amoxicillin is the treatment of choice.

    c Tonsillectomy is of benefit in the long term.

    d Delayed scripts are useful in decreasing the use of antibiotics.

    e Throat swabs should be done in all patients.

96 Regarding the treatment of atopic eczema, which of the following statements is true?

    a Steroid creams should be applied twice a day.

    b Topical antibiotics are required in most cases.

    c Eumovate® is the most potent steroid cream.

    d Reducing the frequency of application of topical corticosteroids reduces their efficacy and risk of local side-effects.

e Once-daily application of topical corticosteroids does not seem to reduce efficacy in comparison with twice-daily application.

97 A 46-year-old gentleman presents with tiredness, polyuria and polydipsia. He is constipated with mild, generalised abdominal pain. Blood test results are as follows. What is the diagnosis?

Fasting glucose	4.8mmol/L	(4.0–7.0mmol/L)
Thyroid stimulating hormone (TSH)	2.1mU/L	(0.3–5.0mU/L)
Free thyroxine	18pmol/L	(9-25pmol/L
Corrected calcium	2.9mmol/L	(2.12–2.65mmol/L)
Phosphate	0.5mmol/L	(0.8–1.5mmol/L)
Parathyroid hormone	75ng/L	(10–60ng/L)

a Myeloma
b Milk alkali syndrome
c Diabetes insipidus
d Primary hyperparathyroidism
e Sarcoidosis

98 Which one of the following is not true about qualitative research?

a Triangulation refers to the process of three independent researchers analysing the same data.

b The validity of a paper is improved by using multiple research methods.

c The iterative process means altering the research methods and the hypothesis over the course of data collection.

d Focus groups and passive observation are useful research tools.

e Inductive reasoning refers to the generation of ideas from data collection.

99 What is the definition of negative predictive value?

  a The proportion of people with a positive test result who do not have the illness in question.

  b The proportion of people with a negative test result who do not have the illness in question.

  c The proportion of people with a negative test result who have the illness in question.

  d The proportion of people with a negative test result.

  e The proportion of people with a positive test result.

100 Which one of the following is not a screening tool for alcohol dependence?

  a EPDS

  b MAST

  c AUDIT ✓

  d CAGE

  e RAPS4

Answers Paper 3

1 a

The Alzheimer's Research Trust has shown a link between aspirin and the slowing in progression of Alzheimer's symptoms, and possibly the prevention of Alzheimer's disease. Beneficial links have also been made with colon cancer. Further research is being undertaken at present. Reference: www.alzheimers-research.org.uk/

2 b

On an ECG the PR interval corresponds with the time taken for excitation to spread from the sino-atrial (SA) node through the atrial muscles and the atrio-ventricular (AV) node down the Bundle of His into the ventricular muscle. A normal PR interval = 0.12–0.20 seconds.

3 b

This is a possible case of leukaemia and hence it is essential to find the cause. Therefore a full blood count, clotting studies, liver function tests and bone marrow aspirate may be indicated. Hepatosplenomegaly is not associated with scurvy or non-accidental injury. HSP is more common in boys and a purpuric rash is mainly seen over the lower extremities and extensor surfaces.

4 e

eGFR (estimated glomerular filtration rate) is an estimate and is found to be least accurate near the normal level. In Afro-Caribbeans, the eGFR must be multiplied by 1.21 to get an accurate value.

5 c

Type II infection recurs more often than Type I and typing may be useful in patient counselling. Reference: Sen P, Barton SE. Genital herpes and its management. *BMJ*. 2007; **334**: 1048–52.

6 d

Economic analysis is used to define choices in resource allocation. It takes into account direct, indirect and intangible costs. Cost/benefit analysis measures the outcome in monetary units and cost utility analysis measures outcomes in quality adjusted life years (QALYs).

7 c

Immobility associated with more than 3 hours' continuous travel in the month before surgery increases the risk of DVT as do: obesity; malignancy; taking hormone replacement therapy or the combined oral contraceptive pill; varicose veins; previous DVT; previous personal or family history; inflammatory bowel disease; recent MI/stroke, etc. Reference: http://guidance.nice.org.uk/CG46

8 a

Seretide® = fluticasone and salmeterol

9 b

NICE 2005 Urgent referral guidelines for suspected upper gastrointestinal cancer include: patients of any age with dyspepsia and iron-deficiency anaemia, as well as patients aged over 55 years with unexplained recent onset dyspepsia.

10 c

Primary adrenocortical insufficiency causes Addison's disease, affecting the glucocorticoid, mineralocorticoid and sex hormone axes. Usually the cause is autoimmune-mediated destruction of the adrenal cortex. Clinical features of Addison's include muscle weakness, hypotension, anorexia, weight loss, reduced pubic and axillary hair and depression. Reference: www.gpnotebook.co.uk

11 d

12 i

13 l

14 a

Mode = number repeated the most in the list of values given (20)

Mean = average of all values (47)

Median = number in the middle of the list when all values are placed in numerical order (30)

Range = the highest value minus the lowest value in the list (103)

15 b

Twenty per cent of women aged 75–85 years have severe osteoporosis. By the age of 70, about a third of Caucasian women will have at least one osteoporotic vertebral fracture. The incidence of osteoporosis is highest in Caucasian women. About 20% of women aged 90 will have had a hip fracture. The incidence of femoral neck fracture increases markedly after the age of 65 years, by the most in Caucasian women. The incidence of vertebral fracture increases markedly after the age of 50 years. Reference: www.gpnotebook.co.uk

16 d

Mebendazole is the medical treatment of choice. The eggs can remain infectious for up to 20 days. Therefore, environmental measures play an important role as the eggs can be caught from objects, e.g. clothing, towels, carpets or bedding.

17 c

Causes of AS include: congenital or rheumatic heart disease; bicuspid heart valve, or hypertrophic cardiomyopathy. Symptoms include dyspnoea, angina, syncope and sudden death. Signs include: a slow rising, small-volume pulse; a heaving, undisplaced apex beat with a narrow pulse pressure, and an ejection systolic murmur best heard in the aortic area which radiates to the carotids (the ejection systolic murmur of aortic sclerosis does not radiate to the carotids). ECG shows left ventricular hypertrophy and chest x-ray may show calcification of the valve. As these patients are at risk of sudden death, prompt valve replacement is recommended. For patients with significant asymptomatic AS, treatment is undecided. Endocarditis prophylactic antibiotics are required.

18 b

19 e

It is a live vaccine and is contraindicated in the immuno-compromised, patients who have egg allergy and pregnant women.

20 c

Babies can make eye contact and smile by 6 weeks of age.

21 d

Further investigation is warranted of a smoker who has no obvious signs of an infection with a cough that has lasted more than 4 weeks.

22 a

The Department of Health (2006–2007) has advised that the following patients should be offered annual influenza vaccination routinely: those aged >65 years; residents of long-term care facilities; asthmatics; diabetics; those with anaemia, chronic heart, lung and kidney disease; those with a weakened immune system such as HIV or long-term steroid usage; women who will be pregnant in the influenza season, and children aged 6–59 months. It should also be offered to those people who have close contact with the above patient groups of any age, e.g. nursing-home staff and household contacts.

23 c

BASH recommends the following stepwise treatment of an acute migraine attack:

Step 1 – Oral simple analgesia, e.g. NSAIDs ± antiemetic

Step 2 – Rectal analgesia, e.g. Diclofenac ± antiemetic

Step 3 – Triptans (oral, nasal or subcutaneous)

Step 4 – Combination of either steps 1+3 or 2+3

Opiates are not recommended as nausea is a side-effect. Reference: www.bash.org.uk

24 a

Recommended treatment for chlamydia by the British Association of Sexual Health and HIV (BASHH) is either doxycycline 100mg bd for 7 days (contraindicated in pregnancy), azithromycin 1g stat, erythromycin 500mg bd for 10–14 days or ofloxacin 200mg bd/400mg od for 7 days. Don't forget contact tracing. Reference: www.bashh. org/guidelines

25 i

26 c

27 h

28 e

29 d

30 a

Fibroadenosis is a benign condition typically affecting 20- to 45-year-old premenopausal women. It presents with cyclical breast tenderness and intermittent breast masses or areas of thickening. Examination should be repeated at different stages of the menstrual cycle as the findings invariably change under the influence of hormones. Treatment consists of breast support, mild diuretics, non-steroidal anti-inflammatory drugs and evening primrose oil. Danazol and even surgery are other options in severe cases.

Fibroadenomata are common in 15- to 35-year-old women. On examination, they are very mobile, non-tender, rubbery and smooth to the touch. They are also known as breast 'mouse', and treatment depends on age. If <40 years and diagnosed with ultrasound and fine needle aspiration, excision is not required unless the diameter is >4cm. If <40 years, it should be excised.

Duct ectasia, more common in women in their fifties, is caused by dilatation of the ducts behind the nipple and periductal inflammation causing areolar pain and erythema. Nipple discharge is thick and cream/green in colour. There may be an areolar mass and the nipple may retract after healing with fibrosis. Mammogram is essential. Treatment involves antibiotics if infected, incision and drainage if there is an abscess, or mammodochectomy.

Fat necrosis usually results from trauma to the breast. Fat cells rupture and an inflammatory response causes calcification in the breast tissue. Presentation is with a tender hard lump, which can become irregular and tethered to the skin. Differential diagnosis includes breast carcinoma and hence investigation with fine-needle aspiration (FNA) and mammography may be required.

Breast abscess usually occurs in breast-feeding mothers due to acute mastitis. The patient is usually systemically unwell with fever and anorexia. The breast is warm to touch, with a tender swelling. The abscess may become fluctuant and discharge spontaneously. Antibiotics effective against *Staphylococcus* may be sufficient if given early, but incision and drainage may be necessary.

Breast carcinoma is the commonest malignancy in women. Risk factors include family history, early menarche and nulliparity. Lumps can be painless or painful. Peau d'orange, skin tethering, nipple inversion/discharge and Paget's disease of the nipple may be presenting features as well as supraclavicular or axillary lymphadenopathy. Signs of metastases to bone, brain, lung or liver may also be present. Diagnosis and staging may require FNA, Trucut biopsy, bone scan, liver ultrasound and brain CT. Treatment options vary from wide local excision +/– axillary clearance to radical mastectomy. Radiotherapy and anti-oestrogens such as tamoxifen are widely used in primary or recurrent disease.

31 c

http://www.dh.gov.uk/en/Publicationsandstatistics/Publications/PublicationsPolicyAndGuidance/DH_065946. There is also a published summary on the RCGP website. Licence to practise must be renewed every 5 years. Specialist recertification applies to GPs as well. Appraisal will include summative components. *All* doctors will undergo revalidation. The appraisal process will *not* lose its formative components.

32 a

NICE Hypertension guidelines 2006 recommends that patients younger than 55 years be treated with an Angiotensin Converting Enzyme (ACE) inhibitor as first line with the addition of a calcium channel blocker or a diuretic if further treatment is necessary. www.nice.org.uk

33 e

Inflammatory bowel disease, not IBS. (BNF)

34 e

Guided self-help books have proven beneficial for mild depression. St John's wart has been shown to be of benefit in mild to moderate depression; however, it is not recommended by NICE (2004) due to its interactions with other medications – e.g. the oral contraceptive pill – as well as uncertainty in respect of dose due to variation in strengths of preparations.

35 b

Beware! Infantile polycystic renal disease is less common than adult polycystic kidney disease and is autosomal recessive. Adult polycystic kidney disease is autosomal dominant.

36 b

37 a

Central retinal artery occlusion causes painless loss of vision within seconds, usually due to thrombo-embolism. The retina appears white with a cherry-red spot at the macula. A risky treatment is to press firmly on the globe and when it becomes painful to remove the pressure quickly, which may dislodge the embolus and restore vision. This can only be done within 1 hour of the start of symptoms. Optic nerve atrophy will cause permanent visual loss if the occlusion lasts more than 1 hour.

38 d

A systematic review aims to perform a thorough and critical search of relevant literature on particular studies which must adhere to its criteria. Systematic reviews are not all equal as their criteria may not be strict enough, allowing studies that are weak to be included. This can introduce bias and error into a review. When data from these studies is pooled and statistical analysis applied to it, it is called a meta-analysis. www.evidence-based-medicine.co.uk

39 e

Full maternity leave entitlement prevails in the event of a stillbirth at *24* weeks gestation or if the baby is born alive at any gestation. Reference: www.direct.gov.uk

40 d

Reference: www.resus.org.uk. Ensure you are up to date with new guidelines, which can change.

41 c

Approximately two out of three men with a raised PSA will not have prostate cancer. Reference: www.cancerscreening.nhs.uk/prostate

42 b

Tuberculosis in HIV-positive patients may be difficult to detect. A Mantoux test may be falsely negative and presentation may be atypical. HIV-positive patients also have an increased rate of reactivation of latent TB and a previous BCG vaccination may be of no protection in these patients. A suspicious CXR and/or acid-fast bacilli in the sputum are used as diagnostic markers and patients are only said to be free from TB after at least two sputum cultures are negative for acid-fast bacilli. TB treatment lasts 6 months and is usually coordinated by local TB chest clinics.

43 b

Causes of short stature include: family history, constitutional delay of growth and puberty and growth hormone insufficiency. Turner's syndrome is relatively common with 1 in 2500 female live births being affected. In pre-school years, approximately 25% of affected girls will be of normal height. In addition to a wide carrying angle and webbed neck, inverted widely spaced nipples and multiple pigmented naevi, eustachian tube dysfunction, progressive sensorineural deafness and strabismus are also common. These children have a normal IQ.

44 k

45 b

46 i

47 c

48 g

49 k

50 b

51 e

Reference: http://www.britishairways.com/travel/healthmedcond/public/en_gb

52 c

Due to reports of blood dyscrasias and liver cirrhosis with methotrexate, the Committee on the Safety of Medicines has advised that a full blood count, renal and liver profiles should be checked before treatment starts and repeated weekly until therapy is stabilised. Monitoring should then take place every 2 to 3 months. Advice should be given to report a sore throat, unexplained bruising or mouth ulcers (symptoms of blood disorders), nausea, abdominal pain or dark urine (i.e. symptoms of liver disease) and any shortness of breath (i.e. respiratory effects).

53 b

Treatment options for warts include: occlusion for 24 hours a day (e.g. with Duct Tape®); wart paint containing salicylic acid, which works by removing dead surface skin cells, and podophyllin which is a cytotoxic agent. Podophyllin must not be used in pregnancy or women considering pregnancy. Seventy per cent of warts will resolve with the use of wart paint, but it may take up to 12 weeks. Cryotherapy also has a 70% success rate after 8–12 weeks of regular freezing.

54 b

The blue needle is used to administer the vaccine intramuscularly. Contrary to popular belief, the smaller needles actually can cause more skin reactions than the larger ones if they are used for intramuscular vaccinations. Diggle L *et al.* Effect of needle size on immunogenicity and reactogenicity of vaccines in infants: randomised controlled trial. *BMJ.* 2006; **333**: 571.

55 d

Approximately 1 in 25 adults in UK carry the cystic fibrosis (CF) gene. It is inherited as an autosomal recessive inheritance pattern. If two carriers meet, the risk is one in four children having CF. That is $1/25 \times 1/25 \times 1/4 = 1/2500$.

56 b

Metabolic syndrome is associated with truncal obesity, high triglyceride levels, raised plasma fasting glucose, raised blood pressure and low HDL levels. Total cholesterol levels are not used to diagnose the syndrome, which is a collection of risk factors for ischaemic heart disease. Insulin resistance is thought to be the underlying cause. For full diagnostic criteria see www.gpnotebook.co.uk

57 d

Under the Ottawa rules for x-ray of ankle injuries, an x-ray is indicated if one of the following is present: pain over the posterior edge of either lateral or medial malleolus; pain at the base of the 5th metatarsal or navicular bone, as well as the inability to weight bear immediately after injury.

58 c

Other sequelae include: ectopic pregnancy; pelvic inflammatory disease (PID), and tubo-ovarian abscess. The perihepatitis caused by *Chlamydia* is called Fitz-Hugh Curtis syndrome. Cervical cancer is associated with human papilloma virus. Ovarian cancer, which is associated with infertility, may also have an association with PID/*Chlamydia* infection; however, as yet there is no hard evidence proving this.

59 b

If symptoms such as polyuria, polydypsia and unexplained weight loss are present, the diagnosis of diabetes mellitus requires a random venous plasma glucose level ≥ 11.1mmol/L; a fasting plasma glucose level ≥ 7mmol/L; or a plasma glucose concentration ≥ 11.1mmol/L, 2 hours after a 75g glucose load in an oral glucose tolerance test (OGTT). If asymptomatic, a confirmatory venous sample is required. Capillary blood glucose levels, HbA1C levels and the detection of glycosuria are not diagnostic. www.who.int

60 d

According to NICE guidelines for COPD (February 2004), COPD can be diagnosed when spirometry results show a FEV1/FVC ratio of <0.70 and FEV1 is less than 80% of predicted.

61 c

62 a

63 a

A Med 3 form is white and a Med 5 form is pink. A Med 4 form comes in a booklet with a green cover.

64 a

NICE guidelines state that AF should be confirmed first if symptomatic/asymptomatic with examination /ECG/24-hour tape. Risk factors for stroke should then be taken into account and anticoagulation with either warfarin or aspirin is recommended. AF is either paroxysmal, persistent or permanent. Paroxysmal AF requires rhythm control. Permanent AF requires rate control. NICE advises rhythm control first for patients with persistent AF who are symptomatic, <65 years old, presenting with lone AF for the first time, whose AF is secondary to a treated or corrected precipitant or those with congestive cardiac failure. Rate control is advised first for patients with persistent AF who are >65 years old, with coronary artery disease; those in whom anti-arrhythmic drug use is contraindicated, and those unsuitable for cardioversion, e.g. structural heart defects/previous failed attempts. Reference: http://guidance.nice.org.uk/CG36

65 a

Recommended treatment by the British Association of Sexual Health and HIV (BASSH) for uncomplicated anogenital infection with *N. gonorrhoea* in adults is either ceftriaxone 250mg im stat OR cefixime 400mg po stat OR spectinomycin 2g im stat. Alternatively, ciprofloxacin 500mg po stat OR ofloxacin 400mg po stat can be used. Ampicillin 2g with 1g probenecid po stat may also be used but is a weaker choice. Reference: http://www.bashh.org/guidelines

66 j

67 b

68 e

69 a

70 f

Overfeeding is common in bottle-fed babies. On average, newborns require 100mls/kg/day, increasing to 150mls/kg/day in babies over a week old. Initially, babies feed on demand, eventually settling into a routine of feeding approximately every 3 to 4 hours. By the age of 12 months, a child will feed about 80mls/kg/day.

Epididymo-orchitis may be acute or chronic and can be caused by mumps, gonorrhoea and coliform infection. Painful, swollen red testes are common and usually accompanied by fever. To distinguish from torsion, surgical exploration may be required. Supportive treatments along with antibiotics are indicated.

Intussusception is the invagination of a portion of intestine into its lumen. The peak incidence is between 6 and 9 months of age and commonly occurs in otherwise healthy children. The child presents with vomiting and colicky abdominal pain (draws his legs up and goes pale with an attack of colic). A late sign is blood or mucus in the stool (redcurrant-jelly stool). There may be a palpable, sausage-shaped mass in the abdomen. Diagnosis is made with abdominal x-ray or ultrasound scan. Pressure from a contrast enema may treat the condition, but surgical reduction may be necessary.

Pyloric stenosis occurs in 7 per 1000 births with a 6:1 male:female ratio. It usually presents in babies 3–6 weeks old with progressive non-bile-stained projectile vomiting. The child tends to be hungry after vomiting. The child may be underweight with visible peristalsis in the left upper quadrant and a pyloric tumour is palpable between the umbilicus and right costal margin. Abdominal ultrasound can demonstrate the hypertrophied muscle of the pylorus. A metabolic alkalosis requiring correction with intravenous rehydration is usually required prior to surgical treatment (Ramstedt's operation – pyloromyotomy).

Testicular torsion is a surgical emergency and infarction is a real risk. In torsion, the testis and epididymis twist on the spermatic cord.

It is more common with undescended or 'clapper bell' testes. Clinical presentation is with sudden onset of pain in the testes radiating to the abdomen accompanied by vomiting. The testis is usually swollen, red and drawn up on the affected side. Differential diagnosis includes epididymo-orchitis, torsion of the testicular appendage (hydatid of Morgagni), strangulated hernia and testicular trauma. Surgical exploration and fixation of the testis is vital to preserve it. Infarcted testes must be removed as auto-antibodies which could lead to infertility may develop.

71 e

Recommended first-line antibiotics are trimethoprim 200mg bd for 3 days or Nitrofurantoin 50mg/100mg qds for 3 days. http://www.hpa.org.uk/infections. This is an excellent resource to use when revising and has valuable information presented in a concise manner.

72 c

Finasteride is an inhibitor of 5-alpha reductase in the testosterone metabolism pathway, which reduces prostate size and lowers PSA. This makes it difficult to interpret the PSA result when using it as a screening tool or to monitor cancer treatment.

73 d

Those with a past history of ischaemic heart disease, the elderly and women tend to delay seeking help. From the BHF fact file *Delays in Treatment for Acute Myocardial Infarction*, November 2006. Reference: www.bhf.org.uk/factfiles

74 d

Recurrent stroke risk is high (30–43% within 5 years), therefore early secondary prevention is a priority in this group of patients. The ESPRIT trial (aspirin plus dipyridamole vs aspirin alone after cerebral ischaemia of arterial origin) was a randomised controlled trial which showed that the addition of dipyridamole slow release (200mg bd) to aspirin reduced the risk of recurrent stroke. From the December 2006 edition of the British Heart Foundation factfile, *Early Intervention in Stroke*. Reference: www.bhf.org.uk/factfiles.

75 a

Post-splenectomy, *Streptococcus pneumonia*, *Haemophilus influenzae* type b, Meningitis C and Influenza vaccination are required. Life-long prophylactic penicillin is recommended (erythromycin if allergic). Both a medical card and medical alert bracelet should be carried by the patient. The card should detail, amongst other things, what vaccines the patient has had, as well as which antibiotic prophylaxis he or she is taking.

76 d

A delayed hypersensitivity reaction involving sensitised T-lymphocyte cells, taking more than 12 hours to evolve.

77 b

NICE advises the following groups of postmenopausal women to take oral bisphosphonates in the secondary prevention of osteoporotic fragility fractures:

- Women aged >75 years – DEXA unnecessary
- Women aged between 65 and 74 years if DEXA confirms osteoporosis.

In postmenopausal women aged <65 years, oral bisphosphonates are recommended by NICE if:

- DEXA scanning shows a very low bone mineral density, **OR**
- They have osteoporosis confirmed on DEXA **and** one or more of the following age-independent risk factors: BMI<19, family history of maternal hip fracture <75 years, untreated premature menopause, prolonged immobility or the presence of a chronic illness associated independently with bone loss, e.g. rheumatoid arthritis.

78 d

Associated with truncal obesity and development of diabetes, fatty liver infiltration is a common cause of abnormal liver test results. Usually, the transaminase levels are elevated, but with an AST:ALT ratio <1 and a normal MCV. Fatty liver disease may progress to cirrhosis and rarely, liver failure.

79 d

Gardasil® is a vaccine against the Human Papilloma Virus (HPV), effective against subtypes 16 and 18 which cause 70% of cervical cancers, and against subtypes 6 and 11, which along with 16 and 18 cause 90% of cases of genital warts. It is most effective if given to girls before they become sexually active. A three-injection course over 6 months is given intramuscularly in the deltoid region.

80 d

A recent study suggests wet combing with conditioner using the 'Bug Busting Kit' gave better results than the use of other over-the-counter remedies. When considering chemical treatment, lotions, liquids or cream are preferred to shampoo. Hill N *et al.* Single blind, randomised, comparative study of the Bug Buster kit and over the counter pediculicide treatments against head lice in the United Kingdom. *BMJ.* 2005; **331**: 384–7.

81 d

82 f

83 p

84 a

85 g

86 n

Missed miscarriage is characterised by a lack of, or mild, symptoms and a uterus smaller than expected. Refer for an early pregnancy scan. Management can be conservative with early pregnancy unit follow-up, or surgical in the form of evacuation of retained products of conception.

Placental abruption (separation of part of the placenta from the uterus) is more common in smokers and after 20 weeks' gestation. PV bleeding does not always occur. Symptoms and signs include those of shock, a 'woody' hard uterus, absent fetal heartbeat or distress on the cardiotocograph (CTG) and abdominal pain which is constant (back pain if the placenta is posterior). Prognosis depends on the size of the separation and the amount of bleeding.

A benign tumour of trophoblastic origin causes a hydatidiform molar pregnancy. No fetal material is present. Choriocarcinoma is the malignant sequela which develops in 1 in 30 cases. Presenting signs/symptoms are PV bleeding, hyperemesis gravidarum, hypertension, and a large uterus for dates. Immediate referral to the gynaecology team is necessary. Ultrasound shows a typical 'snowstorm' appearance. Affected women are followed up by a designated specialist centre. Pregnancy is avoided for a year.

An ectopic pregnancy results from the implantation of the fertilised embryo outside the uterus, mostly in the fallopian tube. The most common presentation is at around 7 weeks' gestation. The risk is increased with an intrauterine device in situ, smoking, a history of pelvic inflammatory disease, blocked tubes or previous ectopic pregnancy. Levonorgestrel, the progesterone-only emergency contraceptive pill, can impede the intra-tubal migration of the fertilised ovum and may increase the risk of ectopic implantation. PV bleeding does not always occur. Abdominal pain may be vague. Diaphragmatic irritation from internal bleeding causing shoulder tip pain is another symptom. Ectopic pregnancy is the leading cause of maternal mortality in the first trimester. Immediately refer to hospital for specialist management, options for which include: expectant (monitor serum β-HCG, may fail spontaneously and resorb), medical (methotrexate) or surgical (salpingostomy/salpingectomy). Subsequent pregnancies should always be referred for early scanning.

Uterine rupture can occur at the site of weakness in the uterine wall, e.g. at the site of a Caesarean section scar. It is uncommon and usually presents with maternal shock and either fetal distress or no audible fetal heartbeat. Risk of fetal death is high. Refer immediately.

Pyelonephritis can occur in up to one-third of untreated UTI cases in pregnancy, increasing the risk of miscarriage. Treatment is aggressive and may necessitate referral for intravenous antibiotics.

87 a

88 b

TMJD is worse as the day progresses. An ESR should be checked if the patient has unilateral pain in order to rule out temporal arteritis. Forte V. Diagnostic genius – temporomandibular dysfunction. *Doctor*. 19 June 2007.

89 b

Eyelid hygiene is the treatment of choice. The eyelids are bathed with a flannel soaked with warm water for 5–10 seconds to soften the skin. They are then massaged to help push out any mucus-like fluid. Finally the eyelids should be cleaned with a cotton wool bud soaked in baby shampoo diluted with warm water in a 50:50 solution. This should be done twice a day until symptoms settle, then once daily to prevent flare-ups.

90 e

Road traffic accidents (RTA) cause the highest number of deaths in children in England and Wales. Fire is also a leading killer of children between the ages of 1 and 4 years. The government has pledged new resources to reduce death rates due to RTA by 2010. This was published in the White Paper *Saving Lives: Our Healthier Nation* 1999.

91 e

Part FF allows for consent to be obtained and signed for by the relevant parties for any body part or tissue to be kept for medico-legal reasons.

92 a

NICE Heart Failure Guidelines 2003 give advice on monitoring beta-blocker usage. They should be started at a low dose and the dose doubled not less than every 2 weeks. Urea, creatinine and electrolytes should be monitored 1 to 2 weeks after the initiation and final titration of dose.

93 b

A white blood cell count (WBC) >50 × 10^9/L, bulky organomegaly/lymphadenopathy, central nervous system involvement and male sex are all factors indicating a worse prognosis in acute lymphoblastic leukaemia.

94 b

NICE 2004 Depression guidelines state selective serotonin re-uptake inhibitors (SSRIs) are the treatment of choice in the elderly. Treatment should be given for a minimum of 6 weeks before assessing efficacy.

95 d

Most sore throats are self-limiting whether due to viral or bacterial infection. If required, phenoxymethylpenicillin is the first-line treatment of choice. It is important not to prescribe amoxicillin, because if the tonsillitis is a presentation of glandular fever, amoxicillin will cause a maculopapular rash. If three or four of the following Centor criteria are present, there is a 40–60% chance of the patient suffering from Group A ß-haemolytic Streptococcus and antibiotics may be beneficial. These include: tonsillar exudate; tender anterior cervical lymph nodes; absence of cough; and history of fever. www.gpnotebook.co.uk

96 e

According to a 2007 *BMJ* review paper, once-daily application of topical corticosteroids in the treatment of inflammatory episodes of atopic eczema does not seem to result in loss of efficacy and could lead to a reduction in local side-effects and cost as well as being more convenient for the patient. Topical antibiotics are not required in most cases. The mainstay of treatment is regular emollients and topical steroids. Dermovate® is the most potent steroid. Williams H. Established corticosteroid creams should be applied only once daily in patients with atopic eczema. *BMJ*. 2007; **334**: 1272.

97 d

Clinical features can include polyuria, thirst, weakness, vomiting, bone pain, pathological fractures, renal calculi and rarely, acute pancreatitis.

98 a

Qualitative research, although statistically weaker than quantitative research, is still extremely useful in general practice. As this type of study looks into hypotheses that may be dependent on people's thoughts and feelings, it may be necessary to alter the research method, known as the iterative process, to reflect this. Triangulation refers to more than one researcher independently analysing the data gathered.

99 b

a = false positive
b = false negative

100 a

EPDS = Edinburgh Postnatal Depression Scale
MAST = Michigan Alcohol Screening Test
AUDIT = Alcohol Use Disorder Identification Test
CAGE = Cut down, Annoyed, Guilty, Eye opener
RAPS4 = Rapid Alcohol Problems Screen Test

Paper 4

1 Which of the following statements is true about mitral regurgitation?

 a It can be caused by endocarditis.

 b It causes a loud S1 heart sound.

 c It always causes left ventricular failure.

 d It is a systolic murmur best heard at the left sternal edge.

 e It is always associated with atrial fibrillation.

2 What part of the cremation form must be completed by the registered medical practitioner who attended the deceased during their last illness?

 a B

 b C

 c D

 d E

 e F

Choose the likely diagnosis from the following list for each clinical scenario below (Questions 3 to 6). Each option may be used once, more than once or not at all.

   a Acute lymphocytic leukaemia
   b Chronic lymphocytic leukaemia
   c Multiple myeloma
   d Acute myeloid leukaemia
   e Chronic myeloid leukaemia
   f Polycythaemia rubra vera
   g Myelodysplasia
   h Non-Hodgkin's lymphoma
   i Hodgkin's lymphoma

3 A 40-year-old male non-smoker presents with a 6-week history of cough and night sweats. On examination, non-tender peripheral lymphadenopathy is noted and the chest is clear on auscultation. A chest x-ray reveals a mediastinal mass and no Reed-Sternberg cells are seen on histological examination.

4 A 3-year-old boy presents with pallor, lethargy and recurrent mouth infections. On examination, he has tender lower legs, splenomegaly and multiple bruises of differing ages.

5 A 58-year-old woman presents with back pain for some time with no preceding trauma. Blood test results show the following:

Haemoglobin	10.3g/dL	(11.5–18.0g/dL)
Urea	15mmol/L	(2.5–6.7mmol/L)
Creatinine	250μmol/L	(70–150μmol/L)
Calcium	3.0mmol/L	(2.12–2.65mmol/L)

6 A 50-year-old man complains of intractable itching mainly after a hot bath. Recently he has also been bothered with recurrent gout. Examination reveals a slightly enlarged spleen.

7 Further assessment is indicated if a child has not acquired the ability to walk unsupported by what age?

a 9 months

b 12 months

c 14 months

d 18 months

e 24 months

8 The treatment of choice for mild to moderate acne rosacea is:

a Topical hydrocortisone 1%

b Metronidazole topically

c Erythromycin orally

d Tetracycline orally

e Solaraze® cream

9 For which of the following patients is human varicella zoster immunoglobulin (VZIG) recommended following contact with chicken pox?

a Bone marrow transplant recipients

b Neonates whose mothers develop varicella within 5 days before or 7 days after delivery

c Neonates born at fewer than 34 weeks' gestation who have been exposed to varicella

d HIV-positive patients

e Patients who have had high-dose steroids 6 months ago

10 Which one statement is not true about Practice-based Commissioning (PBC)?

a Savings from PBC can be spent on patient and non-patient care.

b Practices not taking up PBC will receive the same funding as those practices taking up PBC.

c Tariffs ensure that there is no incentive to bargain on price.

d PBC gives doctors flexibility to tailor the services to their own community.

e General Medical Service (GMS) contract ensures a direct enhanced service (DES) for PBC.

11 According to the November 2006 NICE guidelines for dementia, which of the following drugs are recommended to be used specifically for the primary prevention of dementia?

a Statins

b Hormone replacement therapy

c Non-steroidal anti-inflammatory drugs

d Vitamin E

e None of the above

12 Which one of the following medications is not used in glaucoma?

a Beta-antagonists

b Alpha-agonists

c Prostaglandins

d Mitotics

e Mydriatics

13 According to NICE guidance, which one of the following statements is not true about blood-level monitoring of patients taking Angiotensin Converting Enzyme (ACE) inhibitors?

a Some increase in potassium, urea and creatinine is to be expected.

b A >50% increase above baseline in creatinine is acceptable.

c An increase in potassium to <5.6mmol/L is acceptable.

d If creatinine or potassium rise above acceptable levels then it is advised to halve the dose and recheck the bloods.

e If potassium levels >6.0 mmol/L or creatinine increases by >100% then the ACE inhibitor should be stopped and specialist advice sought.

Match the most likely diagnosis from the list with the clinical scenarios (in Questions 14 to 27). Each option may be used once, more than once, or not at all.

a Tennis elbow

b Golfer's elbow

c Olecranon bursitis

d   Ganglion

e   Trigger finger

f   Dupuytren's contracture

g   Rheumatoid arthritis

h   Osteoarthritis

i   Psoriatic arthropathy

j   Reiter's disease

k   Gout

l   Colle's fracture

m   Smith fracture

n   Dermoid cyst

o   Cyst

p   Polymyalgia rheumatica

q   Bicep's tendon rupture

r   Rotator cuff tear

s   Adhesive capsulitis

t   Bicep tendonitis

u   Supraspinatus tendonitis

v   Carpal tunnel syndrome

w   Scaphoid fracture

x   De Quervain's tenosynovitis

14 A 35-year-old secretary presents with pain over the outer aspect of her right elbow. She states the pain is worse when typing or carrying shopping.

15 A 27-year-old skate boarder presents after a fall with a painful wrist. On examination, you notice a weak grip and pain over the anatomical snuff box.

16 An 18-year-old presents with a painless lump over the back of his wrist.

17 A 40-year-old male presents complaining of 'locking' of his ring finger, which only straightens passively.

18 A 56-year-old known rheumatoid arthritic presents with an acutely swollen non-tender elbow. You notice a soft swelling that is compressible over the ulnar surface of the elbow that seems to be attached to the underlying bone.

19 A 62-year-old woman presents with swelling and stiffness over her distal interphalangeal joint.

20 A 34-year-old male presents with a non-tender lump over his biceps region that appeared when exercising.

21 A 72-year-old man presents with the inability to abduct his shoulder actively, which occurred after trying to hang up a picture. You can abduct his shoulder.

22 A 32-year-old primigravida presents at 34 weeks with pins and needles over both her thumbs and first fingers. It is worse at night and relieved by running cold water over her wrists.

23 A 54-year-old woman presents with the inability to move her shoulder. On examining her shoulder, there is loss of both active and passive movements.

24 A 46-year-old lady presents with painful swollen proximal interphalangeal joints of both hands with weakness in her grip. She informs you that she has recently suffered from a painful red eye that was treated with steroid eye drops for 6 weeks.

25 A 50-year-old man presents with pain in his elbow. On examination, there is pain on resisted pronation.

26 A 55-year-old diabetic presents with thickening over his palm. On examination, he is unable to extend his ring finger.

27 A 40-year-old woman complains of pain in her wrist after gardening. On examination, the radial styloid is tender.

28 According to the March 2006 NICE guidelines for tuberculosis (TB), which one of the following statements is a criterion for neonatal BCG vaccination?

a The neonate is born in an area where the notification rate of TB is 25 per 100 000.

b There is a family history of TB within the last 10 years.

c The mother visited a high-incidence country in the last year.

d There is a family history of TB within the last 3 years.

e The neonate is born in an area where the notification rate of TB is >40 per 100 000.

29 A 55-year-old man presents with a fever and malaise. On examination, his temperature is 39 °C, the pulse is 94 beats/minute and of regular rhythm, and a systolic murmur is heard. Which one of the following investigations would not be useful in diagnosis and treatment?

a Urinalysis

b Blood cultures

c Exercise tolerance test

d Chest x-ray

e Echocardiography

30 A randomised controlled trial of 500 patients comparing lisinopril to placebo shows that there is an absolute risk reduction (ARR) of 5% in the incidence of stroke in the treatment group. What is the number needed to treat (NNT)?

a 5

b 15

c 20

d 10

e 0.05

31 What is the recommended first-line investigation for menorrhagia according to the January 2007 NICE guidelines?

a Serum ferritin

b Thyroid function tests

c Oestrogen levels

d Full blood count

e Serum iron

32 According to current UK Resuscitation Council Guidelines, what is the optimum ratio of compressions to breaths when administering basic life support?

a 15:1

b 15:2

c 30:1

d 30:2

e 25:2

33 An asthmatic patient is currently using a salbutamol inhaler and 400mcg/day inhaled beclometasone. He is still troubled by breathlessness on exertion and also a night-time cough. According to the British Thoracic Society guidelines, what is the most appropriate management?

a Daily oral steroids

b Addition of theophylline tablets

c Introduction of montelukast

d Addition of salmeterol

e Increase beclometasone to 800mcg/day

34 Which one of the following primary cancers does not commonly metastasise to the brain?

a Breast

b Testes

c Lung

d Prostate

e Lymphoma

f Stomach

g Malignant melanoma

35 With reference to the 2006 NICE guidelines on inhaled insulin, which one of the following statements is correct?

a Inhaled insulin is a routine treatment option for sufferers of Type I and Type II diabetes.

b Inhaled insulin should not be used during pregnancy.

c GPs may commence inhaled insulin therapy in diabetic patients who exhibit needle phobia or have significant problems with injection sites.

d Inhaled insulin is made from porcine insulin.

e Inhaled insulin should not be used if no improvement is seen in the HbA1C level after 3 months.

36 A GP is called to see a 2-year-old child at home. He has a fever and has been vomiting since the morning. On examination, he is febrile with a temperature of 39 °C, has cold peripheries and is sleeping. He has a non-blanching spot on his ankle. What is the first thing that you would do?

a Set up intravenous access for fluid resuscitation.

b Prescribe an antipyretic.

c Refer to the on-call paediatric team.

d Prescribe an oral antibiotic.

e Administer intramuscular benzylpenicillin.

37 According to the Quality and Outcomes Framework (QOF) how often must a patient with coronary heart disease have his blood pressure recorded?

a Every 6 months

b Every 9 months

c Every 12 months

d Every 15 months

e Every 18 months

38 What is one of the recommended treatments for pyelonephritis according to the Health Protection Agency?

a Ciprofloxacin 250mg bd for 14 days

b Co-amoxiclav 625mg tds for 14 days

c Ciprofloxacin 500mg bd for 14 days

d Co-amoxiclav 325mg tds for 14 days

e Amoxicillin 500mg tds for 14 days

39 Which of the following is a normal body mass index (BMI)?

   a 12

   b 22

   c 27

   d 32

   e 35

40 Which of the following drugs do not cause gynaecomastia?

   a Spironolactone

   b Cimetidine

   c Methyldopa

   d Marijuana

   e Frusemide

   f Ketoconazole

41 Which of the following statements is not true of subchondral haematoma?

   a Prophylactic antibiotics are necessary to prevent infection.

   b Usually caused by trauma causing shearing of the perichondrium from the underlying cartilage.

   c Should be drained and packed.

   d Packing should be removed after 7 days.

   e Mis-management can result in a cauliflower ear.

42 Regarding maternity leave, when should an employee inform her employer of her pregnancy and the amount of maternity leave she wishes to take?

   a At least 4 weeks before the expected week of confinement

   b At least 6 weeks before the expected week of confinement

   c At least 15 weeks before the expected week of confinement

   d At least 20 weeks before the expected week of confinement

   e At least 25 weeks before the expected week of confinement

43 Concerning *Helicobacter pylori* infection, which one of the following statements is true?

a   Serology testing is useful to distinguish between current and past infections.

b   'Test and Treat' is of no benefit in un-investigated dyspepsia.

c   Blood serology testing is better than stool antigen testing when distinguishing between past and current infections.

d   Breath testing apparatus can be prescribed on FP10 forms.

e   When carrying out the breath test it does not matter if a patient is currently on a proton pump inhibitor at the same time.

44 Concerning Type 2 Diabetes mellitus, which one of the following statements is true?

a   Blood pressure control is important in reducing cardiovascular mortality.

b   Control of blood sugar is the most important risk factor for prevention of cardiovascular disease.

c   High blood pressure and microalbuminuria should be treated with thiazides as first-line treatment.

d   There is no need to treat high lipid levels.

e   Sulphonylureas are first-line treatment of choice for blood glucose control.

45 The first-line treatment for severe Post Traumatic Stress Disorder is:

a   Counselling

b   Selective serotonin re-uptake inhibitor (SSRI) medication

c   Psychotherapy

d   Debriefing, especially after catastrophes

e   Cognitive Behavioural Therapy (CBT)

46 A 6-year-old boy presents with a subconjunctival haemorrhage in his right eye. He has been suffering from a cough that has been getting worse over the past week. What is the most likely diagnosis?

   a Non-accidental injury

   b Pertussis

   c Viral conjunctivitis

   d Measles

   e Rubella

47 A 68-year-old gentleman presents with large blisters over his body which appear to be flaccid. You are told by the patient that they rupture easily. What is the most likely diagnosis?

   a Pustular psoriasis

   b Pemphigoid

   c Pemphigus

   d Allergic reaction

   e Wagner's granulomatosis

Match the following investigations to the clinical scenarios below (in Questions 48 to 52). Each option may be used once, more than once or not at all.

   a Full blood count

   b Thyroid function tests

   c Fasting lipids

   d ECG

   e 24-hour blood-pressure monitoring

   f 24-hour ECG

   g Exercise tolerance test

   h Angiography

   i Thallium scan

   j Echocardiogram

48 A 35-year-old anxious woman presents with a history of palpitations for 2 months. On examination, her pulse rate is 94 beats/min of regular rhythm and she displays a fine tremor.

49 A 50-year-old male smoker presents with chest tightness on climbing the stairs. On examination the blood pressure is 150/92mmHg and chest is clear.

50 A 62-year-old woman presents for the second time with palpitations. Previous blood test results were all normal. On examination, the heart sounds are normal and the heart rate is 72 beats/min of regular rhythm.

51 A 46-year-old woman presents with central chest pain on going up stairs. She has been very tired recently and notes her periods have become longer and heavier. On examination, her pulse rate is 97 beats/min of regular rhythm, blood pressure is 110/70mmHg, heart sounds are normal and her lung fields are clear on auscultation.

52 A 5-year-old child is brought to the GP with fever, cough and vomiting. On examination, the child has a runny nose and a temperature of 38.2 °C. A pure diastolic murmur can be heard. There is no cyanosis.

53 Which one of the following is not a cause for short stature?
a Neglect
b Growth hormone deficiency
c Hyperthyroidism
d Cystic fibrosis
e Hypothyroidism

54 According to *BMJ Clinical Evidence*, what is the first-line treatment for community-acquired pneumonia?
a Amoxicillin for 7 days
b Penicillin V for 7 days
c Clarithromycin for 5 days
d Cephalexin for 7 days
e Amoxicillin for 5 days

55 Which one of the following statements is correct about chlamydia?

    a Does not present with post-coital bleeding.

    b Is asymptomatic in up to 80% of men.

    c Is asymptomatic in about 80% of women.

    d Complications of chlamydia cost £10 million in the UK annually.

    e Genital infection is caused by *C. psittaci.*

56 What is the WHO definition of osteoporosis in terms of bone density measurement?

    a T score >1

    b T score <–1.5

    c T score <–2

    d T score <–2.5

    e T score >–2

57 Which one of the following statements is true regarding acute infective conjunctivitis?

    a Conjunctivitis in children under 1 month is a notifiable disease.

    b Chloramphenicol is the treatment of choice and should be prescribed from the start.

    c Good eye hygiene plays no part in the management.

    d Children should be excluded from school.

    e There is a classic 'cobblestone' appearance of the upper eyelid.

58 In these times of increased demand for patient access, telephone consulting is on the rise. The actual content of a conversation between two people is estimated to represent how much of its total value?

    a 50%

    b 40%

    c 30%

d 20%

e 10%

59 A 26-year-old in her first pregnancy consults you complaining of hearing loss. She states that she hears better in noisier environments. You notice she has blue sclera and her tympanic membranes are normal. What is the diagnosis?

a Bilateral impacted wax

b Chronic otitis media

c Otosclerosis

d Eustachian tube dysfunction

e Tympanosclerosis

60 A 52-year-old overweight banker presents with sudden onset left-sided abdominal pain, and constipation. The pain is worse on movement. He has a slight fever with mild left iliac fossa tenderness but no organomegaly and no guarding. He has not been travelling recently. Observations are normal. What would be your further management?

a Prednisolone enemas

b Oral rehydration only

c Admit for intravenous fluids and antibiotics

d Mesalazine

e Oral cephalexin and metronidazole

61 According to NICE hypertension guidelines, what is the next most appropriate treatment option for a 60-year-old African male who is on amlodipine but has a sustained blood pressure of >160/60mmHg?

a Change to ramipril

b Add in ramipril

c Change to bendrofluazide

d Add in atenolol

e Change to losartan

62 Which one of the following statements is not true of Med 5 certificates?

   a Can be used if it has been more than 1 day since the patient was seen.

   b A certificate should not cover a forward period of more than 4 weeks.

   c A doctor has not seen the patient but on the basis of a written report 5 weeks ago from another doctor can issue a certificate.

   d Can be used if a 'closed' Med 3 certificate was not given previously.

   e Is pink in colour.

63 Which one of the following is an example of autosomal recessive inheritance?

   a Friedrich's ataxia

   b Ehler's–Danlos syndrome

   c Down's syndrome

   d Noonan's syndrome

   e Colour blindness (red-green)

64 Which one of the following statements is not true about smoking cessation pharmacotherapies according to the British Thoracic Society?

   a Pregnant women can use Nicotine Replacement Therapy (NRT).

   b Scientific evidence suggests combining different forms of NRT is not beneficial.

   c There is no specific indication for NRT usage rather than bupropion

   d NRT is available on a NHS prescription

   e Long term usage is not recommended

65 Concerning anti-obesity medication, which of the following is not a centrally acting drug?

   a Ritalin

   b Rimonabant

   c Sibutramine

d Orlistat

e Thyroxine

66 With respect to tennis elbow, the most effective and long-lasting treatment is:

a Local steroid injection

b Physiotherapy

c Non-steroidal anti-inflammatory treatment

d Intramuscular diclofenac

e Wait-and-see approach

67 According to the new NICE guidelines on treating hypertension, what is the first line treatment for an Afro-Caribbean male aged 45?

a Angiotensin Converting Enzyme (ACE) inhibitors

b Beta blockers

c Calcium channel blockers

d Angiotensin receptor type 2 inhibitors

e Mannitol

68 Which of the following tumours has its peak incidence in men aged 20–30 years?

a Testicular seminoma

b Testicular teratoma

c Testicular lymphoma

d Testicular mixed seminoma-teratoma

e Testicular dermoid

69 Regarding the antibiotic ciprofloxacin, which one of the following statements is false?

a It is recommended for the treatment of pneumonia in a child.

b It may cause tendonitis, and lead to tendon rupture.

c It is active against chlamydia.

d The dose for treatment of gonorrhoea is a single 500mg dose.

e It is a licensed treatment of both inhalational and gastric anthrax.

70 A 28-year-old presents with nocturia, polyuria and polydipsia. Urine dipstick is normal and blood tests confirm a slightly raised serum sodium level. What is the diagnosis?

    a Cushing's disease

    b Diabetes insipidus

    c Diabetes mellitus

    d Conn's syndrome

    e Syndrome of Inappropriate Anti-Diuretic Hormone Secretion (SIADH)

Match the nerves listed with their respective roots (in Questions 71 to 76). Each option may be used once, more than once or not at all.

    a C5, C6, C7, C8, T1

    b C7, C8, T1

    c C1, C2, C3

    d L4, L5, S1, S2

    e S1, S2, S3

71 Tibial nerve

72 Ulnar nerve

73 Common peroneal nerve

74 Median nerve

75 Radial nerve

76 Sciatic nerve

77 Which one of the following drugs is not associated with the development of gout?

    a Thiazides

    b Omeprazole

    c Sulphonamides

    d Alcohol

    e Salicylates

    f Frusemide

78 British Hypertension Society guidelines recommend aspirin for primary prevention if the 10-year cardiovascular risk >20% and if the blood pressure is above:

a 130/80mmHg

b 130/85mmHg

c 140/90mmHg

d 145/95mmHg

e 150/90mmHg

79 Which one of the following milestones would you expect a normally developing 10-month-old infant to have most recently acquired?

a Pulling to stand

b Sitting unsupported

c Transferring hand to hand

d Rolling from prone to supine

e Rolling from supine to prone

80 Which one of the following is not a risk factor for developing pre-eclampsia?

a Multiple pregnancy

b Change of partner

c First pregnancy

d Smoking

e Diabetes

81 According to the British National Formulary, the initial treatment dose of prednisolone for polymyalgia rheumatica is:

a 5–10mg orally once a day

b 10–15mg orally once a day

c 15–20mg orally once a day

d 20–30mg orally once a day

e 30–40mg orally once a day

82 Erysipelas is usually caused by:

a *Clostridium difficile*

b *Staphylococcus aureus*

c *Streptococcus aureus*

d *E. coli*

e *Streptococcus pyogenes*

83 Which one of the following statements is not true of B-natiuretic peptide?

a It is independent of the severity of left ventricular function and prognosis.

b It is a neurohormone secreted by myocytes.

c It allows differentiation between cardiac and respiratory causes of breathlessness.

d It is an inexpensive test.

e Should be used in conjunction with an ECG for diagnosis.

84 A 31-year-old gentleman presents with tiredness, weight gain and dry skin. You notice an enlarged thyroid gland and slow relaxing reflexes. Blood test results show the following. What is the diagnosis?

Free thyroxine (T4)	10.1pmol/L	(9–24pmol/L)
Thyroid stimulating hormone	13.31mU/L	(0.3–5.0mU/L)
Thyroglobulin antibody titres	low	
Anti-thyroid peroxidase antibody titres	raised	

a De Quervain's thyroiditis

b Hashimoto's thyroiditis

c Grave's disease

d Myxoedema

e Toxic multinodular goitre

85 According to NICE guidelines 2005, which one of the following symptoms does not require an urgent referral for suspected lower gastrointestinal (GI) tract cancer?

a New symptom of either rectal bleeding or change of bowel habit (looser) for 6 weeks or more in a patient over 60 years of age

b Palpable rectal mass or right abdominal mass

c Aged 40 and over with both blood in the stools and increased bowel habit for 6 weeks or more.

d Unexplained iron-deficient anaemia

e A feeling of incomplete evacuation and intermittent left iliac fossa pain in patients aged 40 or more

86 Concerning computerised Cognitive Behavioural Therapy (CBT) and the treatment of depression, which of the following programmes is recommended by NICE?

a Fear Fighter

b Try for Happier Times

c Depression Understood

d Beating the Blues

e Mood Gym

87 Which one of the following is a natural preventer of stone formation in the urinary tract?

a Phosphate

b Citrate

c Cysteine

d Oxalate

e Urate

88 Which of the following immunisations has been added to the current childhood immunisation schedule?

a Pneumococcal vaccine at 2, 4 and 13 months of age

b Pneumococcal vaccine at 2, 3 and 4 months of age

c Pneumococcal vaccine at 2, 3, and 12 months of age

d Pneumococcal vaccine at 3, 4 and 12 months of age

e Pneumococcal vaccine at 13 months and 3–5 years of age

89 According to the British Hypertension Society, optimal blood-pressure treatment goal for non-diabetic patients in the secondary prevention of stroke is:

a <130/80mmHg

b <145/85mmHg

c <140/85mmHg

d <135/85mmHg

e <130/85mmHg

90 According to the latest Confidential Enquiry into Maternal and Child Health (CEMACH), thromboembolism or thrombosis is a direct cause of what proportion of maternal deaths?

a About 5%

b About 10%

c About 15%

d About 20%

e About 30%

91 What is essential to be checked by a doctor prior to signing the cremation form?

a Metallic joints, i.e. hip replacement

b Cerebral metal work, e.g. aneurysm clips

c Prosthetic limbs

d Pacemaker

e False eye

92 Which one of the following is not a recognised risk factor for chlamydia infection?

a Age under 25 years

b Undergoing termination of pregnancy

c Barrier contraception

d Use of the oral contraceptive pill

e New sexual partner

93 In the treatment of Type 2 Diabetes mellitus, which type of insulin has 24 hour action and a low incidence of hypoglycaemia, therefore useful in treating elderly patients?

a Mixtard 30/70 ®

b Insulatard ®

c Insulin lispro

d Actrapid ®

e Insulin glargine

94 Regarding impetigo which of the following statements is true?

a Children should be excluded from school.

b Oral treatment should always be used.

c The causative organism is *Staphylococcus epidermidis*.

d It leaves scarring.

e It is not very contagious.

95 With reference to the 2006 NICE guidelines on the management of urinary incontinence in women, which one of the following statements is false?

a Pelvic floor muscle training should be offered to women in their first pregnancy to help prevent urinary incontinence.

b Duloxetine is recommended as second-line treatment for stress incontinence.

c First line treatment for urge or mixed incontinence is bladder training for at least 6 weeks, once other causes have been ruled out.

d Post menopausal women with overactive bladder symptoms may be treated with topical oestrogens.

e Urodynamic investigations before commencing treatment are not essential.

96 Which one of the following statements is false with regard to Angiotensin Converting Enzyme (ACE) inhibitors according to NICE guidance?

a Dosage should be doubled every week.

b Start at a low dose.

c Aim for the target dose of the medication.

d A small dose of ACE inhibitor is better than no ACE inhibitor at all.

e Monitor renal function and blood pressure.

97 Regarding herpes zoster infection, which one of the following statements is true?

a Aciclovir is most effective if started within the first 5 days of onset of the rash.

b Co-administration of oral prednisolone and antivirals has been shown to reduce pain and speed up the healing of lesions.

c Tricyclic antidepressants are ineffective in established post herpetic neuralgia.

d Aciclovir is given orally at a dose of 400mg twice a day for 7 days.

e The fetus of a pregnant woman is still susceptible to varicella syndrome if the mother has varicella antibodies and is exposed to active herpes zoster.

98 Regarding the management of psoriasis in pregnancy, which one of the following statements is true?

a Calcipotriol is recommended as first line treatment.

b Topical steroids may be teratogenic.

c Ultraviolet B (UVB) therapy is the safest systemic treatment.

d Both men and women should avoid methotrexate for 1 month preconceptually.

e In women retinoids should be avoided for 6 months preconceptually.

99 Regarding the treatment of threadworms, which one of the following statements is false?

a Mebendazole is the treatment of choice in adults and children older than 2 years.

b Piperazine and senna is an alternative treatment and is only licensed for adult treatment.

c Mebendazole needs repeating after 2–3 weeks if re-infection occurs.

d All household members should be treated.

e Environmental and personal hygiene measures are also important.

100 According to NICE Hypertension guidelines 2006, what is the most appropriate first-line treatment for a Caucasian 60-year-old male smoker with a sustained blood pressure of >160/90mmHg?

a Ramipril

b Atenolol

c Losartan

d Amlodipine

e Propranolol

Answers Paper 4

1 a

Mitral regurgitation can be congenital or caused by rheumatic heart disease, chordae tendinae or papillary muscle rupture after a MI or mitral valve prolapse. Symptoms include fatigue and dyspnoea which can progress to orthopnea and paroxysmal nocturnal dyspnoea. Atypical chest pains and palpitations may be a feature. There is a pansystolic murmur which radiates to the axilla. Left ventricular failure and atrial fibrillation may be present. Echocardiography and angiography are used to assess severity. Medical treatment may be needed for pulmonary oedema but surgery (valve replacement or valve repair) is the definitive cure.

2 a

Since Harold Shipman was found to be guilty of murdering his patients for financial gain, legislation and safeguards have been introduced to prevent this recurring. Currently, Parts B and C of the cremation form are signed by two different doctors. Part B is completed by the registered practitioner who attended the deceased during their last illness, i.e. the GP who saw the patient within the last 14 days, or any of the doctors who attended the patient in hospital.

3 h

4 a

5 c

6 f

Non-Hodgkin's lymphoma is a group of lymphomas which are predominantly B-cell proliferations. It typically presents in adults with lymphadenopathy. Fever, weight loss, lethargy and night sweats may also be present. Investigations may show pancytopenia and a mediastinal mass on CXR. Node biopsy is essential and staging may require CT or MRI scanning. Reed-Sternberg cells are present in Hodgkin's lymphoma. Histologically low-grade lymphomas are slow growing but often incurable and the high-grade lymphomas are more aggressive but curable with chemotherapy regimes.

Acute lymphocytic leukaemia (ALL) typically presents in a child aged 2–10 years (peak 2–4 years), more commonly in boys. It accounts for approximately 85% of all childhood leukaemia. There is also a peak incidence in 40-year-old patients. Signs include pallor and dyspnoea from anaemia, infections of the mouth and skin from neutropenia and spontaneous bruising and bleeding from the gums and nose due to thrombocytopenia. Bone pain, hepatosplenomegaly and chest signs are also common manifestations of organ infiltration. Chemotherapy and supportive measures are needed for treatment. Five-year survival rates for childhood ALL≈70% and adult ALL≈30%.

Multiple myeloma usually occurs over the age of 50 years. The sex ratio is equal. Abnormal B lymphoid cell proliferation causes bone marrow infiltration, localised tumours and osteolytic deposits. Patients present with symptoms of bone pain, particularly in the back, femur and pelvis. Signs of anaemia, infections and pathological fractures may also be presenting features. Diagnosis is made on the presence of Bence-Jones proteins on urine electrophoresis and an M-band on serum electrophoresis. The erythrocyte sedimentation rate is greatly increased. Serum urea, creatinine and calcium may also be raised. X-rays show punched-out lesions (pepper-pot skull). Treatment is supportive and includes chemotherapy. Survival rates may be more than 5 years.

Polycythaemia rubra vera (PRV) is a malignancy due to the proliferation of red blood cells which usually occurs in patients over the age of 50 years and has an incidence of approximately 1.5 per 100 000 per year. Presenting signs of hyperviscosity include visual disturbances ('slow-flow retinopathy') and headaches. Angina, Raynaud's phenomenon and an itchy body, especially after a hot bath, are also common. Gout due to increased red-cell turnover may also be a feature. Splenomegaly is present in approximately 60% of cases. Full blood count may show raised Hb (>20g/dL), PCV, WBC, platelets and decreased MCV. Treatment with regular venesection may be necessary. Slow progression to acute leukaemia occurs in 15% and 30% progress to myelofibrosis.

7 d

8 b

Solaraze® cream is used in treatment of actinic keratosis.

9 a

Varicella zoster immunoglobulin (VZIG) is used in certain situations only. These include the immunocompromised, e.g. bone marrow transplant patients or solid organ transplant recipients who are on immunosuppressive medications; patients who have HIV or those on high-dose systemic steroids until 3 months after treatment. Neonates do not have to have VZIG if the mother develops varicella within 5 days prior to and 7 days post-delivery, as they will have maternal antibodies in the system for their protection. Neonates born at fewer than 28 weeks' gestation or weighing less than 1000g may need to be tested for their VZ status as maternal antibodies may not be present.

10 a

Any savings that a practice makes with Practice-based Commissioning must be plied back into patient care only. Practices will be paid the same proportionate amount of money regardless of PBC involvement. Reference: Department of Health website. http://www.dh.gov.uk/en/ Policyandguidance/Organisationpolicy/Commissioning/Practice-basedcommissioning/index.htm

11 e

The recommendation is not to use any of the above for primary prevention of dementia. Reference: http://guidance.nice.org.uk/cg42

12 e

Glaucoma treatment requires miosis of the pupil to allow free drainage of the aqueous fluid.

13 b

NICE heart failure guidelines (2004) give advice on monitoring of ACE inhibitors. Some increase in potassium, creatinine and urea is to be expected on starting an ACE inhibitor. However, an increase of up to 50% in the creatinine level or a level of 200µmol/L, whichever is smaller, is acceptable. An increase in potassium to 5.9mmol/L is acceptable.

14 a

15 w

16 d

17 e

18 c

19 h

20 q

21 r

22 v

23 s

24 g

25 b

26 f

27 x

Frozen shoulder is characterised by pain, stiffness and a limitation of movement of the shoulder, especially external rotation and abduction.

Rotator cuff tear leads to an inability to abduct the arm actively; however, passive abduction is normal. Also, once the arm has been raised above 90 degrees, abduction can be completed due to the action of the deltoid muscle.

Carpal tunnel syndrome exhibits the following clinical features: numbness, paraesthesiae in the hand including thumb, index, middle and radial half of the ring finger. It is more common in pregnancy, obesity, diabetics, rheumatoid arthritis and hyperparathyroidism.

Golfer's elbow (medial epicondylitis) is less common than tennis elbow (lateral epicondylitis). It is characterised by pain across the flexor aspect due to inflammation of the flexor tendons insertion at the medial epicondyle of the humerus.

Dupuytren's contracture is more common in diabetics, alcoholics, and males. There may be a family history. Thickening of the palmar fascia causes restriction in extension of most commonly the ring and little fingers.

De Quervain's tenosynovitis is caused by thickening and inflammation of the tendon sheath containing the abductor pollicis longus and extensor pollicis brevis. Therefore the tip of the radial styloid is tender.

Scaphoid fractures are most common in young adults and are characterised by a fall on an outstretched hand. Signs include anatomical snuffbox tenderness, pain on wrist dorsiflexion and a weak grip.

28 e

Criteria for offering neonatal vaccination according to NICE – the neonate must be born in an area with a TB notification rate of >40 000, OR one or more parents or grandparents born in a high-incidence country, OR there is a family history of TB in the last 6 years. Reference: http://guidance.nice.org.uk/CG33/guidance/pdf/English

29 c

Infective endocarditis must be considered in a patient with fever and a heart murmur. These and haematuria and splenomegaly make up the four cardinal signs. Endocarditis can affect normal heart valves, abnormal heart valves or even prosthetic valves. Causative organisms include *Streptococcus viridans*, *Staphylococcus aureus*, *Coxiella* or *Chlamydia*. Endocarditis can also be non-infective, e.g. with systemic lupus erythematosus. Blood cultures (three sets), urine dipstick, chest x-ray and echocardiography are all essential investigations. Intravenous antibiotics are the treatment of choice though in certain situations valve replacement may also be warranted.

30 c

NNT = 1/ARR = 1/5% = 20

31 d

Reference: http://guidance.nice.org.uk/CG44 NICE states that there is no evidence to do hormonal tests, e.g. thyroid function and oestrogen levels, in the first instance.

32 d

Reference: www.resus.org.uk. You must look this up for the current guidelines.

33 d

Refer to British Thoracic Society Guidelines for full details of step-wise asthma treatment. www.brit-thoracic.org.uk
Step 1 – Inhaled short-acting beta-agonist as required
Step 2 – Add in inhaled steroid
Step 3 – Add in long-acting beta-agonist and assess control
Step 4 – Increase dose of inhaled steroids or consider addition of fourth drug
Step 5 – Daily oral steroids

34 d

Prostate cancer metastasises to the skull and dura. Twenty-five per cent of lung and breast cancers metastasise to the brain.

35 b

Inhaled insulin is contraindicated in pregnancy, poorly controlled asthmatics/COPD and smokers. Treatment can only be initiated by specialists, not GPs, and only for the reasons given in c. It is not a routine treatment for diabetics. Inhaled insulin is made from human insulin. Inhaled insulin use should be discontinued if no improvement in HbA1C is seen within 6 months. Reference: http://guidance.nice.org.uk/TA113/

36 e

This is an obvious case of possible meningococcal septicaemia and hence as a GP, do not waste time calling the paediatric team. The key is to act first with antibiotics and then to ensure safe transport of the child to accident and emergency. Cold peripheries are a worrying but easily missed sign, so ensure that a full examination is performed in all children.

37 d

The following website can be used to find the most up-to-date QOF targets: http://www.nhsemployers.org/primary/primary-890.cfm. Patients with coronary heart disease need to have their blood pressure measured and recorded every 15 months.

38 b

Also ciprofloxacin 500mg bd for 7 days or if susceptible, trimethoprim 200mg bd for 14 days is recommended. If there is no response to oral antibiotics within 24 hours, admit. Reference: http://www.hpa.org. uk/infections

39 b

BMI = weight in kg/height squared in metres = kg/m^2. A normal BMI range is 19–25, 25–30 is overweight and >30 is obese. BMI <18 is considered underweight.

40 e

Other drugs that cause gynaecomastia: verapamil, heroin, captopril, isoniazid, digitalis, phenothiazines, diethylstilboestrol, oestrogens. It is physiological in boys in the neonatal period/puberty. Liver dysfunction, renal failure, trauma, myotonic dystrophy and leprosy are other secondary causes.

41 a

Prophylactic antibiotics are not necessary unless immunocompromised. Cauliflower ear results from the subperichondrial blood collection of the subchondral haematoma overstimulating the perichondrium, resulting in new cartilage and a deformed ear.

42 c

Reference: www.direct.gov.uk. All information regarding employees' and employers' rights and responsibilities is on this website.

43 d

Breath tests should not be done within 4 weeks of antibacterial treatment or 2 weeks of anti-secretory drugs. Both the breath and faecal antigen tests become negative after eradication unlike the serological test, therefore either the breath or faecal test should be used for diagnosis. Treatment with a proton pump inhibitor or 'Test and Treat' are two suggested interventions for un-investigated dyspepsia (NICE 2004). Also guidance suggests that breath test is the best investigation to check for eradication (SIGN).

44 a

The UK Prospective Diabetes Study concluded that tight BP control reduces both macro- and micro-vascular disease in Type 2 DM. Metformin should be used first line to reduce microvascular disease. BHS guidelines 2004 state a patient with Type 2 DM who has high BP and microalbuminuria should be treated with an ACE inhibitor. www.dtu.ox.ac.uk/ukpds

45 e

NICE 2005 states trauma-focused CBT is first-line treatment and should be started within the first month of the traumatic event. Drug treatment is not regarded as a routine option; however, it should be used if the individual prefers not to engage in CBT, or has gained no benefit from CBT, or if there is co-morbid depression or significant hyper-arousal that impairs the individual's ability to benefit from CBT. www.nice.org.uk

46 b

Whooping cough is caused by *Bordetella pertussis* and treatment is essentially symptomatic. Erythromycin is useful in rendering a person non-infectious but does not alter the course of the disease. Children should be kept off school for 5 days after the start of medication.

47 c

Pemphigus is characterised by the formation of blisters within the epidermis while pemphigoid is deeper, at the level of the basement membrane. Therefore the blisters of pemphigus are more fragile.

48 b

49 g

50 f

51 a

52 j

This is likely to be hyperthyroidism as demonstrated by the palpitations and fine tremor. Hence thyroid function tests would be useful.

Male smokers with a history of chest symptoms on exertion should have an exercise tolerance test.

Palpitations are very common and after initial blood tests it is appropriate to organise a 24-hour ECG.

Women with heavy irregular periods can become anaemic. This can cause shortness of breath, palpitations and chest symptoms on exertion.

Heart murmurs in children can be innocent and may present with a concurrent febrile illness. These tend to be systolic in nature. If a child has a diastolic murmur or a murmur that does not settle with the febrile illness, an echocardiogram should be performed.

53 c

Short stature can be caused by child abuse – specifically neglect due to malnourishment – hypothyroidism, cystic fibrosis and growth hormone deficiency.

54 a

Amoxicillin 500mg three times a day is the first-line treatment for community-acquired pneumonia. Erythromycin is to be used in the penicillin-sensitive patient.

55 c

Chlamydia trachomatis is the most common curable STI in Britain. It is asymptomatic in about 70% of women and 50% of men. It can present with post-coital/intermenstrual bleeding, vaginal/urethral discharge, lower abdominal pain or dysuria. Complications of chlamydia cost £100 million in the UK annually. *C. psittaci* causes pneumonia. http:// www.bashh.org/guidelines

56 d

The definition of osteoporosis is a bone mineral density measurement >2.5 standard deviations below the young adult mean – the T score. www.who.int

57 a

Conjunctivitis usually spontaneously resolves in 14 days. Half of infective cases seen in general practice are viral in origin. A recent randomised controlled trial in the *BMJ* suggests that delayed prescribing of topical antibiotics (not to use the prescription for the first 3 days) reduces antibiotic resistance. Everitt H *et al.* A randomised controlled trial of management strategies for acute infective conjunctivitis in general practice. *BMJ.* 2006; **333**: 321.

58 e

(non-verbal = a; paralinguistic = b) This question has been included to highlight the loss of non-verbal communicative value (50%) of a conversation if telephone consulting begins to replace traditional face-to-face consulting. Hence the importance of safety netting is highlighted when consulting by telephone. Car J, Sheikh A. Telephone consultations. *BMJ.* 2003; **326**: 966–9.

59 c

Otosclerosis is worsened by pregnancy and the combined oral contraceptive pill, leading to a conductive deafness as the stapes fixes to the oval window.

60 e

Mild diverticulitis symptoms can be treated with oral antibiotics in the community and referred to hospital if no response.

61 b

NICE Hypertension Guidelines 2006 recommends patients over the age of 55 years or Afro-Caribbeans to be treated for hypertension first line with a calcium channel blocker or thiazide diuretic, then adding in an Angiotensin Converting Enzyme inhibitor if necessary. www. nice.org.uk

62 c

Med 5 forms can be written by a doctor who has not seen the patient but has a report on the patient written less than 4 weeks ago.

63 a

Friedrich's ataxia is an example of an autosomal recessive condition. Ehler's–Danlos and Noonan's syndrome are typically autosomal dominant conditions. Down's syndrome is a chromosomal condition.

64 b

Nicotine replacement therapy (NRT) is the mainstay of helping patients stop smoking. Guidelines from the BTS advise the usage of combinations of NRT in individual cases who may benefit from this. Most pharmacy-led smoking-cessation programmes are run for 4–6 weeks, but it may be necessary for a GP to prescribe NRT on an FP-10 as a longer-term measure for some patients. There are no specific indications for buproprion rather than NRT and hence it is usually after lengthy discussion with the patient that this is started. Remember, caution is needed, especially in patients with a history of seizures. Pregnant women may use some forms of NRT as smoking is considered more harmful to the fetus. www.brit-thoracic.org.uk

65 d

Rimonabant is a cannabinoid receptor antagonist. Sibutramine is a noradrenaline and serotonin re-uptake inhibitor. Orlistat is a lipase inhibitor in the gut, which works by reducing the absorption of fat from the diet.

66 b

BMJ 2006 showed local steroid injections to give the fastest relief from pain; however, this was not sustained long term. Both physiotherapy and a wait-and-see approach were shown to provide the best long-term results, with physiotherapy giving the fastest relief of the two from pain.

67 c

Older patients >55 years and Afro-Caribbeans do not have renin-dependent hypertension, hence first-line treatment is either a calcium channel blocker or a thiazide diuretic. (ACD rule BHS/ NICE guidance.)

68 b

This is more common in men aged 20–30 years. Testicular seminomas peak in those aged 30–40, mixed tumours in those aged 25–35 years, and lymphoma in those aged 60–70. There is no such thing as a testicular dermoid tumour.

69 a

Quinolones are contraindicated in patients with a history of tendon disorders and should be stopped immediately if tendinitis is suspected.

70 b

Diabetes insipidus can either be cranial or nephrogenic in origin; 30% of cranial cases occur after a head injury and lead to confusion or coma due to hyponatraemia.

71 e

72 b

73 d

74 a

75 a

76 d

77 b

Other drugs which may induce hyperuricaemia include: cytotoxics, pyrazinamide and ethambutol. Characterised but not always defined by hyperuricaemia, gout results from a disorder of purine metabolism, which causes urate crystal deposition and painful synovitis. Cartilage damage may occur and large urate deposits are known as tophi. Acute attacks are treated by rest, fluids, stopping any causative drugs and administering NSAIDs, e.g. diclofenac; however, steroids may be necessary. Maintenance treatment includes lifestyle modification, e.g. reducing alcohol intake and making dietary changes, and uricosuric drugs, e.g. allopurinol, which are not effective acutely.

78 e

www.bhsoc.org

79 a

A child will tend to sit unsupported and transfer from hand to hand at 6–8 months. A child may roll from prone to supine at 4 months and supine to prone at approximately 6 months.

80 d

The risk of developing pre-eclampsia is also increased with maternal age <20 years or >40 years; lupus; thrombophilia; hypertension; renal disease; BMI >35; nulliparity, and family history. Smoking and socio-economic status are not risk factors.

81 b

The initial doses are continued until remission of disease activity (monitored by assessment of clinical symptoms and erythrocyte sedimentation rate), then gradually decreased. Treatment may last up to 2 years but relapses are common. In temporal arteritis the starting dose is between 40 and 60mg daily. www.bnf.org

82 e

Rarely may be caused by staphylococci.

83 a

B-natiuretic peptide (BNP) is a neurohormone secreted by myocytes levels of which are measured to diagnose heart failure. It should be used in conjunction with an ECG for diagnosis. It is directly related to left ventricular function and prognosis. In fact, each 100pg/ml increase in BNP relates to a 35% increase in relative risk of death. According to NICE, if BNP levels are normal, it is unlikely that the patient has heart failure. A few new studies have shown that NT-pro BNP may be have a better negative predictive value than BNP and that it may be more useful in patients with concomitant chronic obstructive pulmonary disease (COPD). However, these tests are not widely available in the UK.

84 b

The classical presentation of Hashimoto's thyroiditis is of a hypothyroid patient with a goitre. Immunological investigations show a low titre of thyroglobulin antibodies and high titre anti-thyroid peroxidase.

85 e

www.nice.org.uk

86 d

NICE 2005 suggests a step-wise approach of care in depression. Computerised CBT, watchful waiting, exercise and brief psychological interventions are useful in the management of mild depression. Medication should be introduced to patients with moderate to severe depression. www.nice.org.uk

87 b

Chemicals naturally present in the urine, e.g. citrate, magnesium and pyrophosphate, prevent stone formation. Low levels of these substances can actually increase the risk of stone formation, with citrate being the most important. Calcium phosphate, oxalate, urate and cysteine are types of renal stone.

88 a

The Chief Medical Officer introduced this schedule from 4 September 2006, with a catch-up programme for all children under the age of 2 years. Reference: www.hpa.org.uk

89 c

Patients who have suffered a stroke are at an increased risk of further stroke. BP control should be aggressive. The BP goal in non-diabetics in secondary prevention is <140/85 mmHg and in diabetics who are hypertensive, the optimal goal is 130/80mmHg. http://www.bhsoc. org/pdfs/BHS_IV_Guidelines.pdf

90 e

In the latest CEMACH report, the five commonest causes of direct maternal deaths = thrombosis/thromboembolism (≈30%); followed by haemorrhage (≈17%); death in early pregnancy, e.g. ectopic/ termination/miscarriage (≈15%); hypertensive disease (≈15%) and sepsis (≈11%). Reference: http://www.cemach.org.uk/

91 d

Prior to cremation the initial doctor must check for pacemakers, as they can cause severe damage to the machinery! Metallic parts and even diamond rings tend to cause no damage and come out of the process unscathed.

92 c

Chlamydia is most common in sexually active people under the age of 25 years (prevalence of 5–10% of men and women in this age group). Using barrier contraception regularly is a protective factor. A new partner or more than one sexual partner in the last year increases the risk. http://www.bashh.org/guidelines/

93 e

94 a

Impetigo is a highly contagious superficial skin infection caused by either *Staphylococcus aureus* or *Streptococcus pyogenes*. Topical treatment (e.g. fusidic acid) should be used if the infection is not widespread. Children should be kept off school until lesions are crusted or healed.

95 b

The management of urinary incontinence as advised by NICE involves lifestyle advice, e.g. weight loss, modifying fluid intake and offering pelvic floor muscle training for 3 months in the first instance. Duloxetine is not to be used first or second line routinely for stress incontinence. However, it may be offered as an alternative to surgical treatments. Urodynamic investigations are not necessary before commencing treatment in women with pure stress incontinence. However, if there is a suspicion of detrusor overactivity, urodynamics can be considered. Overactive bladder symptoms in postmenopausal women can respond to topical oestrogens, and this treatment also reduces the incidence of recurrent UTI. Reference: http://guidance.nice.org.uk/CG40/

96 a

NICE heart failure guidelines (2004) give advice about ACE inhibitor usage. It is important to start at a low dose (though high dose may be necessary in some cases) and titrate up slowly – doubling the dose no sooner than 2 weeks after starting. The dose should be titrated to the maximum tolerated or target dose, for example, 10mg ramipril. The electrolytes and renal function should be checked with initiation of the medication and with every increase in dose.

97 b

Herpes zoster, or shingles, is a common condition seen in general practice. It is caused by the reactivation of latent *Varicella zoster* (chicken pox) infection in around 25% of people who have had the infection in the past. Antivirals started within 72 hours of the onset of rash are most effective. These should be given to all those over the age of 50 years with new vesicle formation, or complications whenever they present. Co-administration of prednisolone at 60mg daily, then tapering the dose after 7 days is effective in reducing pain, speeding up lesion healing and reducing morbidity. Tricyclics are effective in reducing the incidence of post-herpetic neuralgia. Aciclovir is given at a dose of 800mg five times a day for 7–10 days (BNF dose). If a pregnant woman has varicella antibodies, her fetus is not susceptible to varicella syndrome if she is exposed to active zoster. From: Wareham D, Breuer J. Herpes zoster: clinical review. *BMJ*. 2007; **334**: 1211–15.

98 c

Psoriasis usually improves in pregnancy and a flare-up may be experienced post partum. First-line treatment includes emollients, topical mild and moderately potent steroids and dithranol, which are all safe in pregnancy. Second-line, systemic treatment which is safest is UVB followed by ciclosporin (both only to be initiated in secondary care). Manufacturers of calcipotriol advise avoidance. UVA is teratogenic. Methotrexate should be avoided 3 months pre-conceptually by both men and women. Retinoids should be avoided for 2 years by women who want to conceive. Reference: Weatherhead S *et al.* Management of psoriasis in pregnancy. *BMJ.* 2007; **334**: 1218–20.

99 b

Piperazine and senna can be used in infants.

100 d

NICE Hypertension Guidelines 2006 recommends that patients over the age of 55 years be treated with a calcium channel blocker as first line with the addition of an ACE inhibitor if further treatment is necessary.

Index

(Q) refers to 'questions'; (A) to 'answers', key concepts or definitions.